FIT FOUNDATION

A GUIDE TO HELP ACHIEVE GOOD HEALTH FOR AMERICA'S OVERWEIGHT YOUTH

10   09   08   07   06   5   4   3   2

Library of Congress Cataloging-in-Publication Data

Schwartz, Harry (Harry Wiesman), 1957-
  Fit foundation : a guide to help achieve good health for ameri-ca's overweight youth / by Harry Schwartz.
        p. cm.
  ISBN 1-56625-266-0
  1. Obesity in children. 2. Obesity in children–Prevention. 3. Children–Nutrition. I. Title.
  RJ399.C6S39 2006
  618.92'398–dc22

                                        2006000398

Cover and Interior Design: Joy Jacob
Cover Photo: Gaku Shiroma
Contributing Photographers: Gaku Shiroma, Susan Bourgoin

Volt Press
9255 Sunset Blvd., #711
Los Angeles, CA 90069
www.voltpress.com

FIT FOUNDATION

A GUIDE TO HELP ACHIEVE GOOD HEALTH FOR AMERICA'S OVERWEIGHT YOUTH

BY HARRY SCHWARTZ

Volt Press
Los Angeles

To Laurie and Alexa, you are my inspiration and you always bring out the best in me.

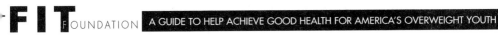
TABLE OF CONTENTS

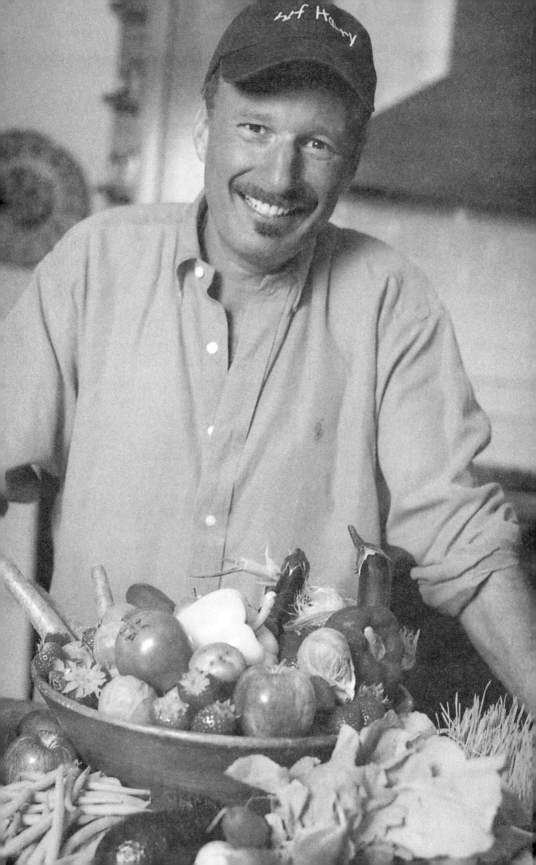

INTRODUCTION

My Story

f I can make one young person get healthier and feel better about him or her self, I will have accomplished what I set out to do. We all have things about our lives and ourselves that we would like to change. Some of those things we have control over and some we do not. This book addresses the ones over which we have some control. Once we understand what we can change and we begin to make these changes, it then becomes easier for us to work through the challenges over which we have little or no control.

From the outside, my childhood looked like a fantasy. My father was very successful, powerful and charitable. My mom is like this combination of Mother Theresa, Auntie Mame, Julia Child and the Make-A-Wish Foundation. My siblings were fine and often fun. I grew up in a

Childhood obesity has reached epidemic proportions. This is the first generation ever that is facing a lower life expectancy than previous generations. While a lot of my inspiration for weight loss stemmed from vanity, this is more about getting healthy and feeling better. A healthy body leads to a healthy mind. I won't kid you, though: a healthy body is also more fun to show off! A natural result of getting fit will be having more confidence in your appearance.

How we feel about and view ourselves affects our self-esteem, productivity and futures. For many, getting fit changes a mindset from wanting to hide to wanting to be noticed. Getting noticed for your accomplishments leads to inspiration. Inspiration leads to motivation. Motivation leads to action. Action leads to results!

mansion with horses, a pool and lots of great cars and toys. We were always going to luxurious and exotic destinations, shopping, having fun, eating great food in great places and laughing. My mom made meals and gave parties that are still talked about decades later.

On the inside, it was a different story. Rather than bore you with personal details, I will simply explain that between my genetics, my reaction to my father's temper and values, some family politics and traditions, and my obsession and weakness with and for food, I was a fat kid. Some eased the label with "husky" or "stocky". I knew I was fat. I hated my body. I was embarrassed by my body. I was uncomfortable with myself. I was ashamed of myself. Fueled by stress, low self esteem, depression and anxiety, I ate more, got fatter and worsened the cycle. I built a wall around myself that limited how I approached every second of every day. I was obsessed.

All through junior high and high school, my calorie intake was extraordinary. My physical activity level was extremely low. There were a few summers when I sweated myself down to husky, but it never lasted. I would start the day with donuts, caramel cinnamon rolls, waffles, pancakes and the like. I always had a double lunch at school. After school snacks included two double cheeseburgers, two large orders of fries and two large colas. I went home from there, snacked some more, and then sat down to meat and potatoes for dinner. There was lots of delicious food available all the time and it was my addiction. Hot fudge sundae or petits fours? The choice was usually both.

By the time I got to college I really don't know what I weighed. It was in the area of 250 pounds. I wore overalls and I could not fasten the side buttons. I could not look in the mirror. I was convinced I was not worthy of a successful life, relationship, career or accomplishment. I was the best my father's money could buy. Who would want to be with me when I did not even want to be with myself? I failed to recognize any positives about who I was because I was blinded by my own fat which disgusted me.

Then, one day, I was getting into the shower and a noise made me turn my head. In that second, I caught a glimpse of myself in the mirror. Full bodied and stark naked, I was face to face with myself. I was right. No amount of black cloth or vertical stripes could help deny it. I was obese. That second changed my life. I lost my appetite. My personal pendulum came to a screeching halt with the first possibility of reversing direction. Ever.

My favorite cousin, Bruce, went to school at the same college as I and he was living with Susan, one of the greatest and most beautiful females attending the college. I loved them both and they loved me. I had a mad crush on Susan but knew that she, or anyone like her, was unobtainable for me.

Eating healthy and living a healthy lifestyle doesn't need to cost more than a fast food and sedentary existence. In fact, in the long run money will be saved on health costs and waste. Shopping at farmers' markets where you can find organic and fresher selections is often less expensive! Getting more active doesn't require joining a gym or health club. It just means choosing to get off the couch.

I think it was Bruce who helped me want to be happy because he had brains, a great sense of humor, looks, toys and the best woman around. He had also been privileged but suffered and survived his own personal battles, been fat and thin, and he was living proof that active, healthy people have more fun. Susan loved food as much as I did and was a great cook. But food was not an obsession with her, it was a passion. That became such an important distinction for me to understand because I really love food and I could never give it up! They both also accepted me for who I was, liked me fat or thin and were instrumental in the process of making me understand that there were things about me worth liking. What a gift they gave me!

Although people noticed a dramatic change in my appearance after my weight loss, to my amazement, most people stated that they never noticed that I was ever that fat. In fact, people who were later asked to describe me as a youth rarely mentioned the fact that I was obese. It obviously has meant more to me than anyone else! This is about *my* self esteem, *my* self image, *my* confidence. And so it is with each of you.

It was up to me to evolve into who I wanted to become. It still is. The problem is that since I was so unhappy with who I was, this evolution has taken a lot of work. I have had a fight on my hands. The enemies have included my habits, my diet, my genes and my own choices. This fight is going to last my entire lifetime. I have had to learn to live with and even love the enemy because, alas, I am the enemy. I have now made peace with the enemy. And so it will be for each and every one of you. This isn't about food. It's about you and me. It's about liking who we are and becoming who we want to be.

Part of who I am is that I love food. I really love food. I love to create it, prepare it, order it, serve it, eat it, drive through and pick it up, smell it, admire it, taste it and experience it. I am talking uncon-ditional love. It was a true sense of joy when I realized that I would *not* have to end my romance with food. I just had to start eating the right things in the right amounts for the right reasons. And I am happier for it. I like being happy. It feels good. There, I said it. And that is just how easy it can be!

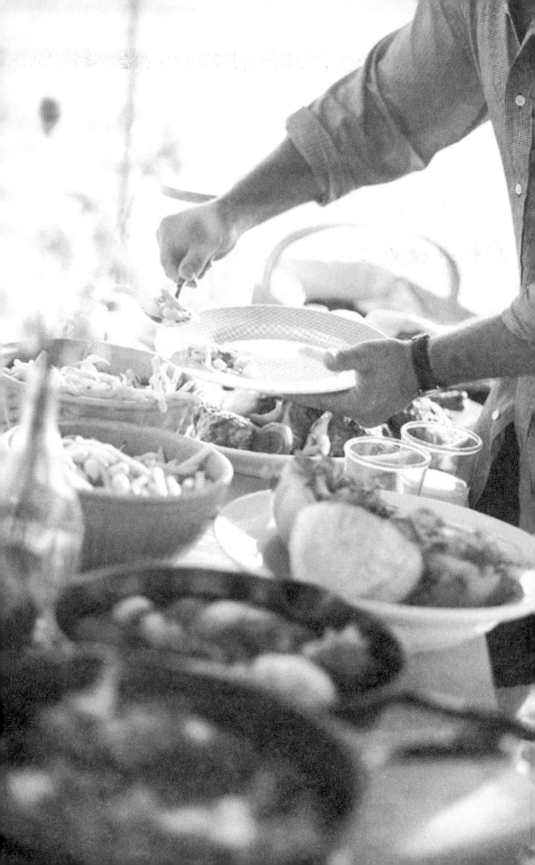

Why We Eat

Choices

We have a lot of choices in life. Choosing to be healthy and lose weight does not have to mean dieting. But making some choices that will lead to a healthy lifestyle can help us lose weight or maintain a healthy weight. I remember a very in-shape, unsympathetic doctor in Dallas who was very insistent that I lose weight, smugly saying, "When it comes to eating, if something tastes good, spit it out because it's not good for you!" That was not only mean and disheartening, it is so untrue. In fact, it made me a little defiant! It also made me want to have a tray of brownies and a milkshake.

I remember the last time I appeared publicly in a bathing suit as a child. I was about seven. Yes, it was forty years ago but I remember that day like it was yesterday. It was

Never say "no" or "you can't" when it comes to eating. Sometimes putting limitations on things makes them even harder to resist. Just make the healthy and nutritious choices available and explain why they are better. Ruining your appetite with a slice of watermelon or cluster of grapes is a good thing!

FIT FOUNDATION tip

Unhealthy high fat or high sugar snacks should never serve as a reward for anything. Food should also not serve as consolation or emotional relaxation. Eat when you are hungry and make good choices based on a healthy balance of nutrition and flavor. After a while, high fat, high sodium and processed foods will not even be appealing.

a hot summer day in Iowa, perfect for swimming at the public pool in Conrad, a small town near where we lived. We went to this pool often in the summer because it was big, new and fun. I loved to jump off the high dive board. I was standing in line to do just that when three older guys appeared from behind me, shoved me and said, "Out of the way, fatso!" I think that was the first time anyone had ever said out loud that I was fat. I may have known it, but no one had ever just put it in my face like that. They might as well have shot me.

I reacted by crying and running back to the comfort of my mother's arms where she, wanting to ease her baby's pain, said, "It's okay honey. You'll grow out of it. Here, have a cookie!!" That pattern of resolving stress, sadness, or conflict by eating had already established itself. The pattern of eating because I was happy or because the sun was out or because it wasn't, and because something looked good or tasted good, or because I was in the mood or just felt like it, had already established itself, too. It also made me want to stay home, stay in, stay covered and watch tv.

I have since talked to my mother a lot about my obesity. She thought she was doing the right thing. From birth, she never let me cry. "I just fed you every time you let out a peep!" she said. Forty years ago there were no segments on the morning shows about obesity and its effects. There were no newspaper articles or magazine features. My mother didn't really connect the fact that what I was eating was making me fat. She was more concerned about my being happy. She didn't even know I was miserable. You were supposed to feed your growing children and eating was giving me pleasure so it must have been a good thing. I was a clone of my round shouldered, obese father and we just thought it was natural. Somehow, I would magically grow out of my baby fat even though he never did. My father had his first heart attack when he was in his early fifties. We now know better.

Having a Fit Foundation does take the whole family. However, it does not take a diet or boring exercise routine. It just takes the desire to be healthy. If you don't want to be healthy, then we need to address that because it could be a reflection of your self-esteem. If you don't want to be healthy and feel good about yourself, then it has to be understood why. If you feel this way and one of the big reasons is because you are obese and feel helpless, we can fix that.

Nothing helped my self esteem more than being healthy, fit and happy with my body. I used to look at the popular guys and shake my head. What would it have been like to be in shape? To have confidence? To wear tight jeans and a tucked in t-shirt? To take off your shirt with confidence and be seen? To have someone have a crush on you? I envied that so much. I used to really get upset about it. So what would I do? I would have a double cheeseburger and fries washed down with twenty-four ounces of sparkling flavored sugar water before supper. Wrong. Wrong. Wrong. Oh what a web we weave when we choose to deceive. And I was deceiving myself. I thought that a snack with enough calories to get me through a day or two would make me feel better.

Today, my family and I eat delicious, satisfying food every day. We eat out, we eat fast food, we go to parties and events and we eat at home. We just make the choices that will not only please our palettes, but that will please our well-being. Also, we don't eat unless we are at least a little bit hungry!

Start at home. When you are filling the refrigerator or pantry, begin by reading some labels. It is amazing what garbage you will find that you have been eating without being aware of it. Here are some very important things to minimize the consumption of just to be healthy. Losing weight will be a by-product of eliminating these unnatural items from our food intake.

(Please note that I am not a doctor or nutritionist. Most of this lifestyle is the result of experience, common sense and a lot of research. Please consult a doctor before dramatically changing any aspect of your lifestyle, especially if you suffer from any medical condition in addition to obesity.)

Trans Fats: Eliminate them altogether. They are the worst kinds of fats, not because of their fat calories but because of their damaging effect on our circulatory system. Even products that claim to be 'all natural' can contain trans fats. This is oil blended with hydrogen. All natural, yes, but studies have shown that this process makes the stuff stick to your veins like glue, which is not a good thing. This has nothing to do with dieting. It is just a good decision for your health. And in doing so, you are going to be forced to steer away from many processed, high fat, unhealthy foods. Good riddance!

Sodium Nitrate and other Preservatives

Studies have shown that Sodium Nitrate and some of its cousin preservatives cause cancer. I don't want cancer if I can avoid it. Let us make the decision to eliminate these for the same reason we eliminated trans fats. In doing so, you will get rid of a lot of fatty, processed, unhealthy meats such as bacon, sausage, salami, pepperoni, bologna, etc. Choose preservative-free lean ham, preservative-free turkey and soy bacon and sausage, and natural smoked turkey products.

Artificial Colors and Flavors Studies have shown some of these artificial ingredients when consumed are danger-ous. Keep away from them for a Fit Foundation.

Salt When healthy, young and active, salt is not that important to watch. Consult a doctor and never overdo the salt, no matter what. I under salt food. You can always add more but it is virtually impossible to remove.

Sugar White, processed sugar may be in a lot of things that taste good but they are really empty calories. Minimize your intake of this and choose natural sugars like fruits, juices, maple syrup and cane juice or non-refined natural sweeteners.

Saturated Fat Here is one that is just common sense. It is the bad kind of fat, so keep away!

Good Choice	Not So Good Choice
Watermelon	Frozen High Sugar Sweets
Frozen Yogurt	Ice Cream
Natural Non Fat Yogurt	Pudding Cup
Angel Food Cake	Cheesecake
Pita Chips	Potato Chips
Salsa	Sour Cream Based Dip
Smoked Chicken Flatbread Pizza	Cheese and Pepperoni Pizza
Lean Ham	Bacon
Smoked Turkey	Processed Cold Cuts
Celery Stuffed with Nut Butter	Crackers and Cheese from a can
Cole Slaw in Vinegar Dressing	Creamy Coleslaw
Grilled Chicken Sandwich	Double Cheese Burger
Ball Game Peanuts	Ball Game Nachos
Fish Tacos	Chimichanga
3 Bean Salad	Potato Salad
Black Beans	Re-fried Beans
Granola Bar	Marshmallow Rice Treats
Spaghetti and Meatballs	Lasagna
Smoked Turkey Roll-up or Wrap	Italian Sub or Philly Cheese Steak
Chicken Noodle Soup	Clam Chowder
Steamed Clams	Fried Clams
Shrimp Cocktail	Shrimp Tempura
Chips and Salsa	Spinach and Artichoke Dip in a Bread Bowl
Pretzels	Potato Chips
Blended Frozen Fruit Drink	Frozen Ice Cream Cookie Treat
Steamed Dumplings	Pan Fried Dumplings
Biscotti	Chocolate Chip Scone

Good Choice	Not So Good Choice
Natural Cheese	Processed Cheese
Soy Breakfast Links	Sausage Patties
Whipped Neufchâtel Cheese	Regular Cream Cheese
Barley Vegetable Soup	Creamy Potato Soup
Baked Pizza Flavored Rice Chips	Fried Pizza Rolls
Fat Free Natural Fig Cookies	Boxed Chocolate Chip Cookies
Low Fat Whole Wheat Crackers	Buttery Boxed Crackers
Grilled Fish Sandwich	Fried Fish Sandwich
Natural Almond Butter	Processed Peanut Butter
Natural Turkey Jerky	Preservative-laden Beef Sticks
Natural Low Fat Ranch Dressing	Mayonnaise
Natural Ramen Soup Cup	Processed Soup
Pasta with Tomato Sauce	Macaroni and Cheese
Frozen Fruit Juice Treat	Ice Cream Cookie Bar
Natural Ginger Snap	Peanut Butter Cookie
Yogurt Covered Raisins	Chocolate Covered Peanuts
Unsweetened Fruit Juice and Club Soda	Grape Soda
Warm Skim Chocolate Milk	Hot Cocoa Mix
Tuna Salad with Low fat Mayo	Ham Salad
Turkey Chili	Fast Food Chili
Black Bean Soup	Bean and Ham Soup
Thin Crust Pizza	Deep Dish Pizza
Soft Tacos with Whole Wheat Tortillas	Crispy Tacos
Small Chocolate Milkshake with Skim Milk	Hot Fudge Sundae with Whipping Cream
An Organic Apple	Sweetened Apple Juice
Pure Maple Syrup	Artificial Maple Syrup
Low or Nonfat Cottage Cheese	Creamy Cottage Cheese
Oatmeal with Maple Syrup	Pancakes with Butter and Syrup

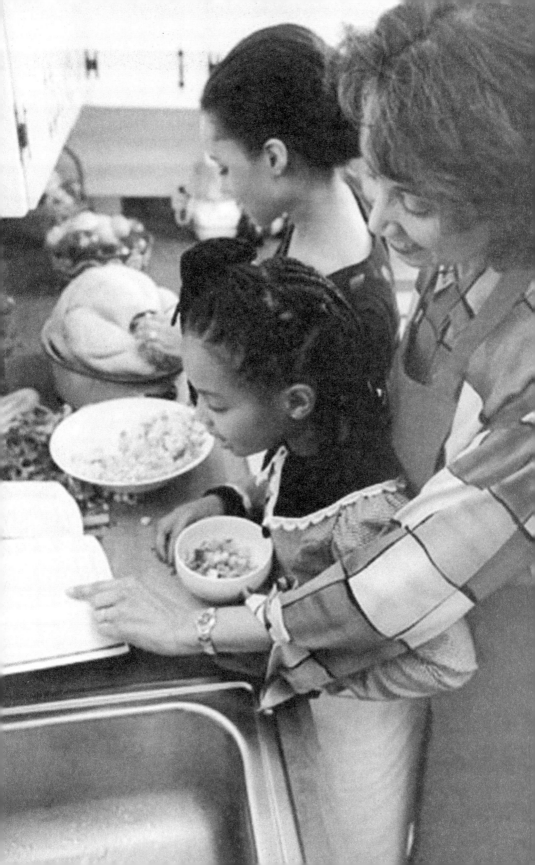

Why We Eat

Genes

Well, **I had finally done it.** I had lost 100 pounds, was taking classes at Harvard, living in a beautiful apartment along the Charles River in Back Bay, Boston, and driving a convertible. I was running 5 miles a day, making the right choices and had met and become engaged to the girl of my dreams. I was wearing 29-inch jeans and feeling pretty darn good about myself and my accomplishments of the last few years.

There is a beautiful clothing store in Boston where I was shopping with my mom for clothes to wear on my honeymoon. I had never been comfortable wearing pleated pants and tailored shirts as I wanted clothes that hung on me to conceal my obesity. At last I was trying on clothes that thin, in-shape guys would wear. But I

Health and fitness are not just affected by diet and exercise but by our genes and family history. We should try and be the best we can be for who we are and not relate it to others or strive to have results that are unreasonable for our own body types. Concentrate on the things you can control. Anything else will lead to frustration and disappointment.

FITFOUNDATION **tip**

Make a game of finding healthy alternatives to sweets, sodas and salty snacks. Sparkling water and orange juice becomes healthy orange soda. Low salt soy nuts and rice crackers make for a great choice over potato chips and peanuts. Making homemade pita chips and hummus is not only healthier but also saves money. Plus, when sharing homemade healthy snacks with friends, you'll feel a sense of pride and accomplishment.

was feeling very insecure. I weighed about 150 pounds and was five foot nine inches, almost underweight. I stood in front of the mirror in the dressing area of the store and was still not very happy with how I looked. I turned to my mom and asked, "Do you think this makes me look fat?"

Before she could respond, a huge man, a perfect stranger who probably weighed 300 pounds who was also in the dressing area, turned to me and said, "Guys like us will never look thin. We have barrel chests and it is just our shape!"

I just stood there feeling like I had in sixth grade. My mother wanted to slap him. I could not even respond. I looked into the mirror and decided that I had definitely changed my body and now it was time to change my mind. I was in good shape and my shape was good. It was time to get happy and secure with myself and I didn't even know how that felt.

I bought those pleated pants and linen tailored shirts and I wore them proudly on my honeymoon with my gorgeous new bride. I snorkeled in my bathing suit and relaxed on the beach of an exclusive resort among the beautiful people and enjoyed every minute. At last I had nothing to hide and I stood proud. To stay that way was still going to take the right choices.

Skip the fries unless you can steal one or two from someone else's plate. Have a baked potato with scallions and plain yogurt or low fat cottage cheese instead of sour cream and butter. Go for the brown rice instead of the white. Choose the vegetable of the day over the mashed potatoes and gravy. Iced tea or fruit-flavored waters over soda and herbal tea over coffee. A hot chocolate made with fat free milk won't hurt you if you are craving something rich and chocolatey. If it's hot out, go for a glass of skim chocolate milk. Put it in the blender with some ice and fat free frozen yogurt and buzz it up for a fat free frappé.

Here are some guidelines when you are eating out or on vacation:

Breakfast

Watermelon, kiwi fruit and berries with yogurt

Whole grain waffles and maple syrup

Scrambled eggs and cheese with scallions and peppers

Poached eggs on an English muffin with strawberries

Whole wheat toast with low fat cream cheese and jams

Crisp flatbread with peanut butter

Granola with a banana and yogurt

Smoked salmon with onions, capers and tomatoes

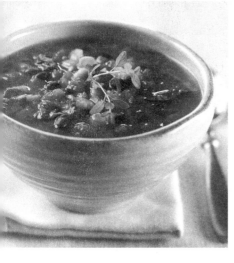

Lunch

Smoked turkey wrap with mustard—hold the mayo

Cobb salad minus the bacon, vinaigrette dressing

Grilled salmon salad

Grilled chicken wrap

Soft chicken tacos

Fish tacos with salsa and guacamole

Stir fry shrimp and veggies

Vegetable soup

Chicken and noodles soup

Tomato soup and a bread stick

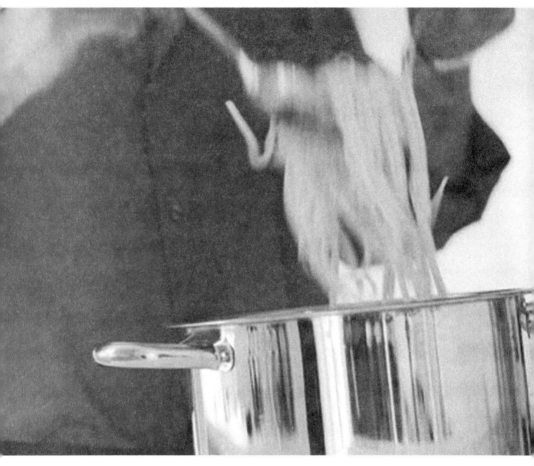

Dinner

Shrimp cocktail

Blackened fish with rice
   and beans

Roasted chicken and veggies

Steamed mussels with herbs
   and tomato

Pasta with tomato basil sauce

Grilled scallops

Lean meat or chicken kebabs

Grilled pork medallions

Steamed dumplings

Fresh summer shrimp rolls

Pad thai with chicken

Mei fun

Braised artichokes

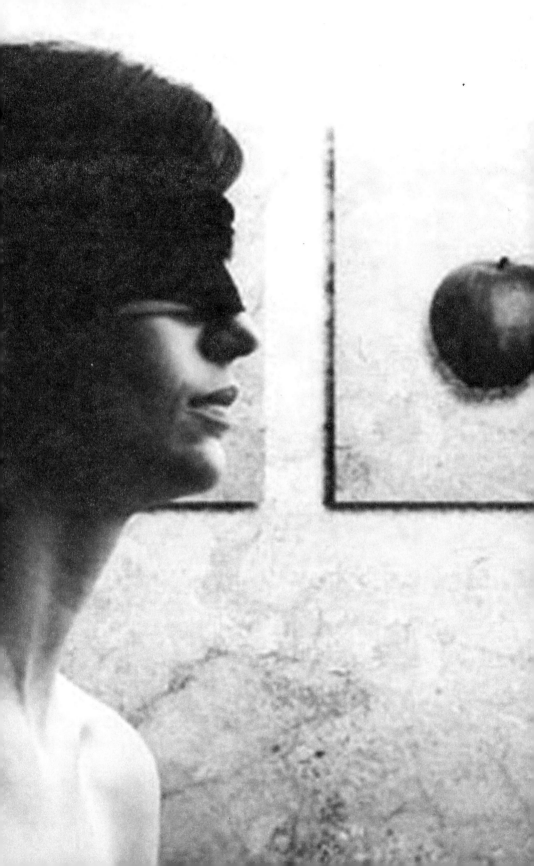

Why We Eat

Addiction

The door to our basement in the house in which I grew up always stirred a contradiction in me. I was scared to go down in that basement. It was cavernous and dark with lots of equipment humming, clanging and blowing. Beyond the cavernous rooms there was a concrete crawl space accessible by a small rectangular opening in which one had to crawl to get around as it was only four feet tall or so. It was really so that plumbing and electrical could be accessed without having to have a full basement. However, if there ever were a bogeyman, he would have lived in the crawl space. There were mousetraps and mice too as it was quite rural where we lived.

On the other hand, behind a door at the bottom of the stairs, under which a troll quite probably lived, there was a treasure. To get to the treasure, one had to

Food can be an addiction, just like drugs, alcohol or cigarettes, and equally unhealthy. Make sure that you are really hungry and for the right reasons before letting anything pass through your lips! If you eat more slowly and take smaller bites, your body will have time to tell your mind that you are full before you have overeaten.

FITOUNDATION

FIT tip

There are healthy sweets and not just fruit and yogurt! Fat free meringue kisses, frozen juice bars, natural licorice bites and fat free sorbet can really kill a craving and satisfy your appetite for desserts without guilt or regret. You will notice in the Sweet Stuff recipe section (p. 161) that many of the recipes use small amounts of butter and sugar. That's OK! When you divide the amounts used by the number of servings, you'll see that it is no big deal. The flavor and nutrition of the fruits and berries far outweighs the small amount of sugar and fat.

brave the stairs and my imagined threats in the basement.

Upon making the dangerous journey, there was a freezer. In this freezer, hidden behind a magic door there was the treasure. Upon opening the freezer door, it was like the lights of heaven were released. I could almost hear angels singing and trumpets heralding.

Besides an assortment of home-baked cookies, brownies and layer bars, there were carrot cakes and chocolate cakes. But the real jewels of the freezer chest were petits-fours from Barbara's Bake Shop in Des Moines. These sweet delicacies were even incredible frozen and I rarely took the time to wait for them to thaw. There I would sit, on a concrete basement floor, in the light from the freezer, beside the humming furnaces, eating what should have been three-bite cakes in one big gulp. I ate them like potato chips. When I think about it now....

That was the price I paid for my mom being one of the

greatest entertainers of all time. The freezer food was really for company but there were no surveillance cameras or inventories taken. The only obstacle between that treasure and me was my fear of the basement. The delicacies in the basement were always worth the risk. I guess if you want to look at the good in any situation, that delicious treasure helped me overcome some fears!

Desserts and sweets aren't inherently bad. I was just guilty of eating for the wrong reasons, eating way too much and making some bad choices. There are some great choices, however, if you want to get and stay fit, even with sweets and desserts. If you are out, choose a small soft-serve ice cream with a bit of chocolate or marshmallow sauce (these are fat free or low fat versus trans-fat laden hot fudge). Have a small chocolate milkshake and ask them to use fat free milk and low fat frozen yogurt. Even a small chocolate bar with almonds is a better choice than a monster cookie or frosted brownie.

At home, have ready to eat slices of watermelon available instead of cookies and cakes. Make or purchase low fat granola squares. Have bowls of rinsed berries ready to pop in your mouth instead of candy. Just make better choices. You don't have to starve or eliminate "the good stuff!"

When I was losing my weight and getting fit, I found a snack that really satisfied me and that I never got tired of. It was quite simple: a butter lettuce leaf with a bit of naturally fat free mayonnaise and some smoked turkey breast all rolled up tightly. It was simple, easy and delicious. Sometimes I had honey mustard instead of mayonnaise. Sometimes I added natural vegetarian

Make deliciously healthy choices available. Instead of a whole watermelon, have small pieces cut up and ready to pop in your mouth. Rinsed berries in a bowl and low fat cheesecake flavored natural yogurts make great snacks. Kids enjoy making melon balls and orange sections. These can be eaten in quantity without a problem. Low fat cheese squares are very nutritious and filling. Making it easy makes it accomplishable.

bacon bits. Occasionally I added a thin slice of low fat cheese. I always kept these things in my refrigerator.

My point is to try and find an easy, quick and healthy snack that satisfies you. Always keep the ingredients on hand. It helps if you can slightly vary it so you don't become bored with it. If it is fast and healthy, you will be less likely to be waiting in line in a fast food joint making a bad choice. After twenty-five years, I still love my lettuce-wrapped smoked turkey. When I think of the calories, time and money I have saved eating my home made "fast food," I can't help but wonder why the world eats so much junk.

And fast food is not really so fast. Waiting in line, waiting to pay, and driving around is a waste of time, gas and energy. Plus, all of the paper and plastic that is wasted is an ecological nightmare. Creating your own quick healthy snacks is not only good for you, it is better for the world!

I am not at all against fast food restaurants as there are now lots of good choices available from yogurt parfaits to grilled chicken sandwiches. When you are out and about at mealtime, these places are great…as long as you make the right choices!

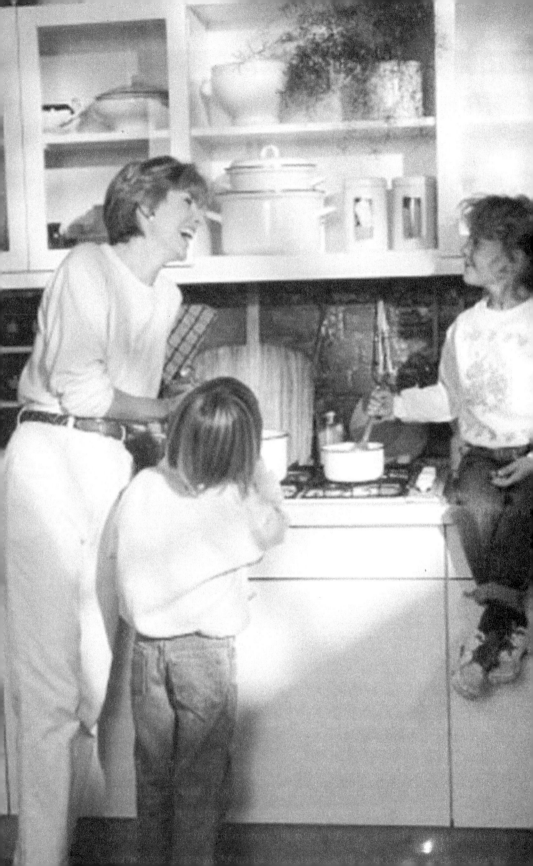

Getting Started
The Method

First, make a commitment to yourself and get a commitment from those around you. This is not a diet. This is not a regimen. This is a lifestyle. Explain to yourself and those around you that you are choosing good health and may need some support. Everyone will want this for you. Most of all, want this for yourself and understand that you *deserve* to be healthy. Take a good look at yourself and imagine what it would be like to be fit. Imagine the clothes you would wear, the things you would do and what it would be like to have that added assurance and self esteem that being fit and healthy would give you. Decide that this is what you want and *go for it*. It really isn't that difficult once you make a decision. You can actually make a game of it. Life is multiple choices. Know that you are going to make the right ones. Add to the following suggested menus a walk with a friend or with your dog, a stroll through the mall, or a bike ride through a safe neighborhood or park, and lots and lots of water.

Getting fit can be fun for the whole family and should involve everyone in the household. The Fit Foundation method does not require starvation or calorie counting. It is just a matter of choice!!!

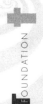

Day 1

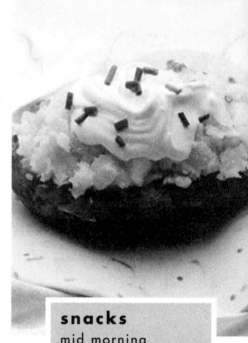

BREAKFAST

1 cup low fat granola mixed into
natural fat free flavored yogurt
1 slice of whole wheat toast with
teaspoon of peanut butter
1 glass skim milk

LUNCH

Smoked turkey roll up with lots of
veggies and mustard, fat free
mayonnaise if desired
Baked tortilla chips and salsa
A glass of chocolate skim milk

SUPPER

A slice of melon
Tossed salad with tomatoes, carrots and
cucumber with a natural low fat Italian
dressing
A grilled chicken breast with salsa
Baked potato with plain yogurt and natural
bacon flavored bits
One half cup frozen low fat yogurt

snacks
mid morning
a banana

afternoon
2 or 3 cups low salt
unbuttered organic
popped popcorn

evening
Avoid this if you can but
if you are hungry, have
a low fat granola bar or
a cup of low sugar cold
cereal with skim milk

Day 2

BREAKFAST
Oatmeal with maple syrup
A bowl of berries
1 glass skim milk

LUNCH
Salad with low fat dressing
Spinach spaghetti with marinara
   sauce and a sprinkle of parmesan
Unsweetened fruit iced tea

SUPPER
A slice of melon
A sliced tomato with a sprinkle of
   low fat mozzarella cheese and some
   low fat dressing
A lean hamburger without the bun, topped
   with grilled or sautéed onions and a
Slice of low fat cheddar cheese
A baked sweet potato or yam with
   a touch of maple syrup
Sparkling water flavored with sugar
   free grape juice
1 cup skim chocolate milk blended
   with 1 cup ice until smooth

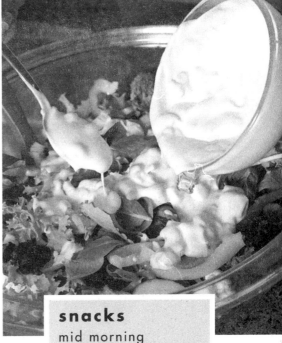

snacks
mid morning
An orange

afternoon
A piece of herbed flat-
bread with some low fat
cheese

evening
Avoid this if you can but
if you are hungry, have
a low fat granola bar or
a cup of low sugar cold
cereal with skim milk

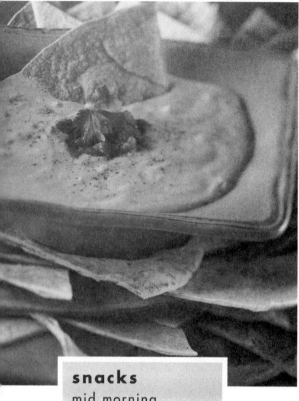

Day 3

BREAKFAST
2 soft boiled eggs
2 slices wheat toast
1 glass skim milk
An apple

LUNCH
Chef's salad with lean meats
    and low fat cheese, low fat
    dressing
Low fat whole grain crackers
Unsweetened fruit iced tea

SUPPER
Baked tortilla chips and salsa
A roasted turkey drumstick
A cup of mashed potatoes mixed with
    roasted garlic and a bit of olive oil
A green vegetable of choice
Sparkling water flavored with unsweetened
    fruit juice
1 or 2 natural ginger snaps

snacks
mid morning
A fat free yogurt

afternoon
2 stalks of celery with 1
tablespoon of natural
peanut butter or low fat
cream cheese

evening
Avoid this if you can but
if you are hungry, have
a low fat granola bar or
a cup of low sugar cold
cereal with skim milk

snacks

mid morning
A fat free yogurt

afternoon
Baked tortilla chips
and salsa

evening
Avoid this if you can but
if you are hungry, have
a low fat granola bar or
a cup of low sugar cold
cereal with skim milk

Day 4

BREAKFAST
A bacon, lettuce and tomato sandwich
made with soy bacon, whole wheat
toast and nonfat mayonnaise
An orange
A glass of skim milk

LUNCH
Tuna salad roll-up made with
nonfat mayonnaise, tomato,
and sprouts
Some low fat or baked potato
chips
A pickle
Unsweetened fruit iced tea

SUPPER
A tossed salad with low fat
dressing
Roasted lean pork roast
Roasted rosemary potatoes
A green vegetable
Sparkling water flavored with
unsweetened fruit juice
1-cup fat free frozen yogurt

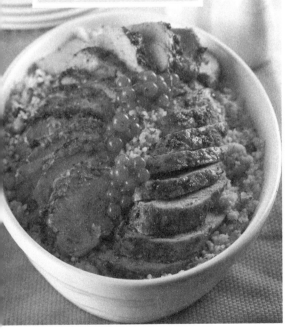

snacks

mid morning
A fat free yogurt or low fat granola bar

afternoon
Pita chips and salsa

evening
Avoid this if you can but if you are hungry, have a low fat granola bar or a cup of low sugar cold cereal with skim milk

Day 5

BREAKFAST
Scrambled eggs with low fat cheddar and scallions
2 slices wheat toast with jelly
A glass of skim milk

LUNCH
Grilled chicken roll-up with veggies and honey mustard
Low fat cole slaw
A few bread and butter pickles
Skim chocolate milk

SUPPER
A slice of melon
Tossed salad with tomatoes and cucumbers with low fat dressing
Hearty beef stew
Sparkling water flavored with unsweetened fruit juice
2 or 3 natural fat free fig cookies

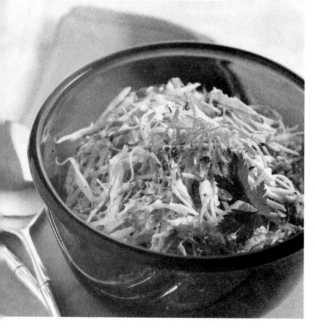

Day 6

BREAKFAST
Yogurt, granola and chopped
   watermelon parfait
Skim milk

LUNCH
A tossed salad with low
   fat dressing
A bowl of chili and crackers
Unsweetened fruit tea

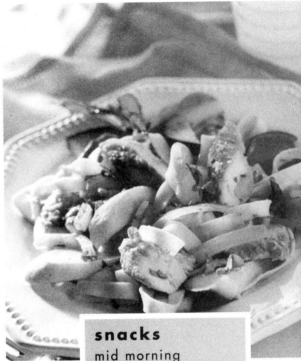

SUPPER
A slice of melon
Pasta with grilled chicken and vegetables in
   garlic flavored olive oil with a sprinkle of
   grated parmesan
Sparkling water flavored with unsweetened
   fruit juice
Frozen low fat yogurt

snacks
mid morning
A banana

afternoon
Carrots and celery with
low fat ranch dip

evening
Avoid this if you can but
if you are hungry, have
a low fat granola bar or
a cup of low sugar cold
cereal with skim milk

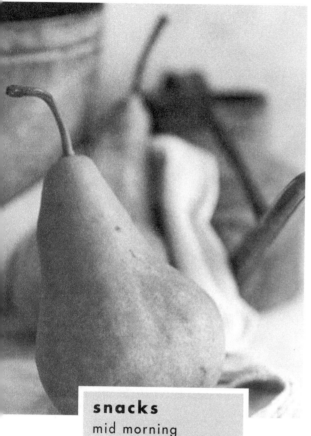

Day 7

BREAKFAST
A piece of fruit
Whole wheat waffles with fruit
or maple syrup
Skim milk

LUNCH
Chicken and low fat cheese
quesadilla with salsa
Unsweetened fruit iced tea

SUPPER
A slice of melon
A tossed salad with cucumber
and tomato with low fat
dressing
Grilled salmon
Roasted bell peppers with
garlic
Sparkling water flavored with
unsweetened fruit juice
Chocolate milk shake made with low
fat ice cream and fat free
chocolate syrup

snacks

mid morning
A fat free yogurt

afternoon
Baked pita chips and
low fat hummus

evening
Avoid this if you can but
if you are hungry, have
a low fat granola bar or
a cup of low sugar cold
cereal with skim milk

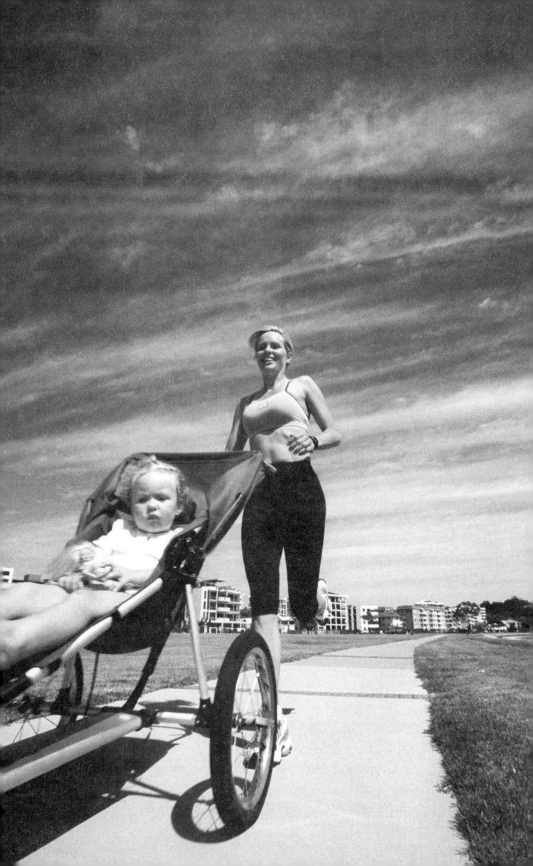

Get Up, Get Going

Getting Fit

eing embarrassed by my body was some-thing I dealt with every day. Until recently, I have not even thought of my health, but focused solely on my appearance. In sixth or seventh grade, much to my horror, it was determined in gym class that the guys would have a basketball game and it would be "shirts vs. skins." When I realized that I was going to have to remove my shirt, I started to hyperventilate. I took control of myself and just did it. I took off my shirt. My head was buzzing and I was light-headed! Then something happened that remains vivid in my mind: I caught my teacher talking to another and it appeared to me that they were pointing and laughing. At me! The worst thing was that I couldn't blame them.

I went running home to my mother. I begged her to convince our pediatrician

Increasing cardiovascular activity not only leads to a healthier body, it leads to a healthier and stronger mental state, outlook and general well-being. Increasing your circulation can positively affect your outlook. Imagine getting healthier and happier at the same time!

Begin slowly when increasing physical activities. Overdoing it with an overzealous beginning and unreasonable goals can lead to injury, disappointment and actually reduce the activities in the long run. It is okay to feel a little soreness with increased activities. But pain is not your friend. If something hurts, stop! A gradual buildup of your activities will reduce any stress on the body and keep your mind looking forward to more activity later rather than dreading the next time.

to give me a doctor's excuse from gym. I got one for the rest of the time I was in Junior High and High School. I, who needed gym class more than any of the guys who were athletic and active, got a doctor's excuse to lie around, burn less calories, get less circulation to my brain and body, be less alert and be less healthy. This was probably not the best decision we could have made. Plus, less activity leads to boredom which leads to, you guessed it, *eating* for the wrong reasons. I was in a vicious downward mental cycle and upward spiraling weight cycle.

My mom was worried about my "happiness" rather than my exercise. I was quite confident that getting out of gym would not only make me happier and reduce some stress, it would all but eliminate my having to expose my body to anyone. I knew I would get teased mercilessly in the locker room and I couldn't deal with that.

The solution should not have been to reduce exercise. The

emphasis should have been on figuring out a way to increase my activity. My mental obsession with the embarassment of my body should have been dealt with right then and there. I should have been encouraged to be more active, even if gym class was not an option for me at the moment because of what was in my head. My continued lack of activity not only affected my physical health, it affected my coordination, my mental health and my socialization with my peers. Perhaps the most damaging effect the sedentary life had on me was in my level of self-confidence.

But enough about me. Like ice cream and french fries, television and computer games are fine—in moderation. It is much more important to get up, get off your rear, get active and get healthy. But organized workouts, overzealous expectations of oneself and starting too fast can be self defeating. The first time I decided to exercise, I ran a few blocks, got a bloody nose and almost passed out. Start walking before you train for a marathon. Get a dog and be responsible for it. You'll have no choice but to go for six walks a day. Go shopping! Yes, walking through a mall is aerobic. Take a few flights of stairs instead of an elevator. Play charades. Make it a game instead of required misery. Just get up and get moving. Here are the ABCs of Fit Foundation activities.

A **Arfing (walking and playing with the dog)** While a family pet is a huge responsibility, it can also be a fun reason to get off the couch and out of the house.

Acting Try out for a play. It is fun, hard work, social and can really increase your confidence and socialization. Plus, it keeps you away from the refrigerator!

Arting Get some water-soluble chalk and make designs on the driveway. Get an easel and canvas and paint the great outdoors. Do a family mural on a wall of the garage or basement.

B **Batting** Play badminton. Play wiffle ball. Play Batman.

Balling Throw a ball to the dog. Play catch with a friend. Bounce a ball off a concrete wall.

Bubbling Get some bubbles and have a contest.

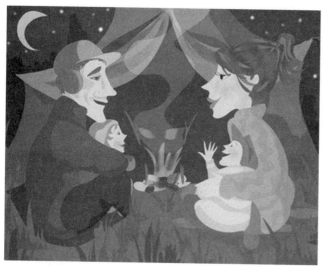

C **Camping** Even if it is just in the great backyard, pitch a tent and forage around. Get outside, play in a treehouse, play American pioneer. Better yet, make the family vacation a camping trip and go for walks and eat what you catch while fishing. Leave the junk food at home and focus on trail mix and turkey or salmon jerky.

Canoeing If you live near an appropriate body of water, get hold of an inexpensive canoe and water safety equipment.

Caroling Not just for the holidays, singing helps us breathe deeper and can be aerobic. Sing in the choir. Sing along with your favorite rapper. Sing in the shower!

D **Dancing** It's okay to watch music videos as long as you dance right along with the music.

Dunking Pushing a ball underwater when you are swim-ming is not only fun but great exercise.

Dressing Make an effort to try on clothes that fit and make you feel comfortable. Shopping and trying on clothes keeps your mind away from the food court and keeps you moving, bending and reaching. You do not have to buy a thing!

E **Earthing** Weed the garden. Plant a tree. Till the earth. It feels great!

Electrifying Cut and hang decorations for holidays, birthdays and celebrations.

Eradicating Clean out the closets, garage and basement. Burn calories, get organized and get rid of the stuff you don't use or need.

Embarking Go on a bike ride.

49

Farming Work out in the country with a friend on the farm.

Fencing Paint or repair a fence, or both. Alternatively, take a fencing class!

Frolicking Roll down a grassy hill. Frolic with a friend in the park.

Folding Take charge of the sheets and towels, folding the laundry.

Giggling Have a good laugh or go to a standup comedy club and make someone laugh.

Garaging Clean out and paint the garage.

Gifting Be in charge of gift wrapping. Keep the supplies organized and put together boxes and wrap for mailing or giving.

Hanging Hang up your clothes and organize your wardrobe.

Hollering Have a dog, cat, pig or sibling calling contest.

Horsing For a lot of us, having a horse or pony is the impossible dream. But if you want one and can have one, it is a great way to get up, get out, get healthy and have fun.

Imaging (Taking Pictures) Take the responsibility for the camera and make a real or digital scrapbook for any event.

Incinerating (Taking care of the trash) Okay, so this isn't too much fun, but it is an activity that needs to be done in every household.

Implementing Start a club and implement a plan to raise some money for a good cause.

J **Jumping** Jumping

rope or hopping on a pogo stick is great and fun exercise.

Jazzing Take up a jazz or jazzercise class.

Juggling Learning to juggle takes a lot of energy and coordination.

K **Kicking**

Kickboxing and kickball are fun and great for you.

Kiting *Go fly a kite!*

Kayaking Learning how to kayak is not just learning a challenging skill, it's fun!

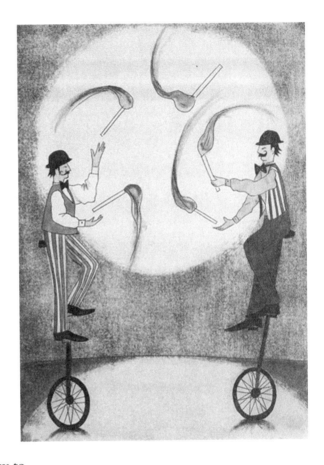

L **Living** Get up, get out, get

fit and enjoy life.

Laundering Collect and do the laundry. It's aerobic and it has to be done anyway!!!

Lassoing Having fun with a rope and a fence post can become addictive. You can have a horseless rodeo in your own back yard!

Literating Join a book club and have your discussions during a walk in the park or along the beach.

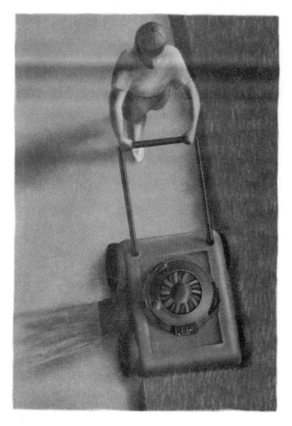

Marketing For your school church or charity organization, sell something door-to-door like magazines or health bars.

N **Nailing** Build something! **Neighboring** Be a good neighbor or grandchild and help out someone with household chores or grocery shopping. **Nurturing** If you are old enough and able to babysit, it is a great way to make money while chasing kids through the house!

M **Mowing** Mowing the lawn and gardening are a great source for burning calories while beautifying the house. Do it for others and you can make some money, too.
Moving Help someone who is moving. Pack boxes or put together the wardrobes.

O **Oaring** Row, row, row your boat.
Organizing Take charge of the books, magazines, family photos, etc. Get them organized and boxed or bound.
Outmaneuvering Set up an

obstacle course and have some fun with friends, family or even a pet!

P **Painting** Paint your room, paint a fence, paint the house, with permission, of course!
Pounding Learn how to play the drums.
Planting Plant seeds, plant a tree, plant a bush and then take care of them.

Q **Quacking** My daughter had a friend who raised ducks. It went from incubation to blue ribbons at the county fair. Great experience. Plus, if you have some fun and walk like a duck and talk like a duck, you'll burn some calories.
Qualifying Try out for something. You might surprise yourself.
Quipping Write and perform

R short stories or poems.
Riding Ride a bike, horse or peddle cart.
Running Start walking first and then work up to a short jog. You'll be amazed how great you feel by the time you are running.
Racketing Tennis and racquetball are awesome exercise and fun!

S **Shopping** There can be a whole lot of walking, pushing, toting and reaching in this activity.
Schlepping Get a wagon and take the groceries from the car to the door.
Showing Put on a talent show.

T **Towing** Get out that wagon again and sell rides.
Tailing Play 'follow the leader.'

53

Treeing Hang a swing from a strong tree limb and get into the swing of things.

U **Un-adorning** Take down and repack decorations.
Undulating Get in the water, extend your arms and move

them back and forth in the water to create waves.
Unwrapping Take the storm windows off the house and wash them.

V **Vacuuming** Vacuum the house, cars or truck.
Volunteering Volunteer to help out at a nursing home or with a sick friend or relative.
Vending Set up an iced tea stand and watermelon wedge stand.

W **Windowing** Wash them until they sparkle!
Washing Take a look at the family car. Could it use a washing?
Walking And walk and walk and walk.
Waltzing Take a ballroom dance class and be the belle of the ball!

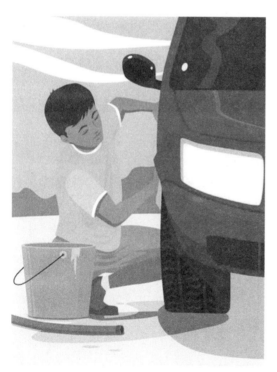

X

X-Manning Go outside and play "X-Men."

X-Raying Play Superman or Superwoman.

X-Cavate Dig a hole and plant a tree, with permission.

Y

Yodeling Climb a hill, yodeling all the way!

Yacht Learn how to sail.

Yarn Learn how to knit.

Yearbook Join the yearbook committee and go in search of great photographs.

Z

Zig-Zag Set up poles and race through them.

Zip Zip around the block a few times.

Zooing Go to the zoo and see it on foot rather than from the train!

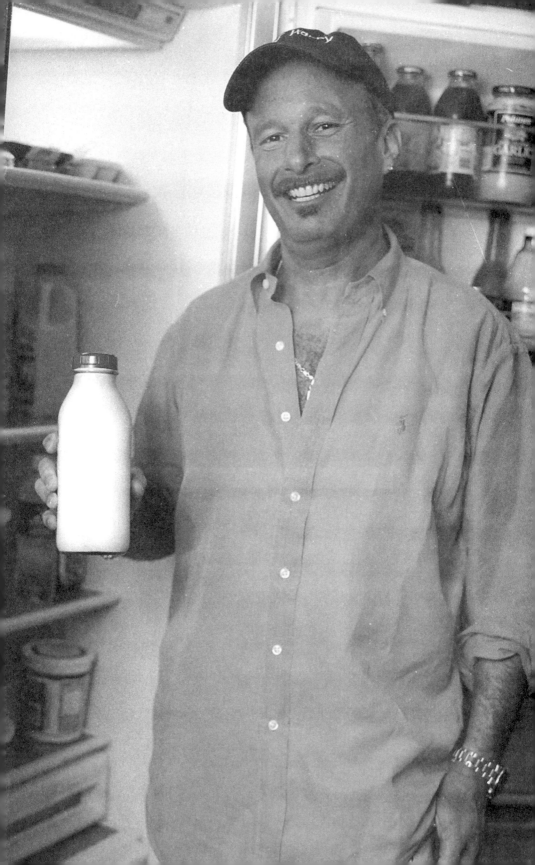

Refrigerator Essentials

It is so important to make it easy to make the right choices. Having things around that are good for you, easy to make and eat and satisfying is essential. A bag of washed lettuce and a low fat natural dressing, cut up fruit, sliced smoked turkey, salsas and baked chips, low fat hummus, spelt bread or whole wheat wraps, non-fat chocolate milk, fat free yogurt and natural sugar-free jams should be staples in your Fit Foundation kitchen. Plus, there are lots of creations you can make yourself. And you'll have fun doing it. Make cooking aerobic. Walk to the store, unpack the groceries, shake your dressing in a tightly closed jar and shake your body at the same time. Just have fun making the right choices and it is easy to be fit!

It is very frustrating when you are hungry or ready to cook only to open a refrigerator and find nothing of interest. Many condiments and dairy products have long shelf lives and should always be on hand. Determine what you use often and keep these things well stocked.

FIT FOUNDATION tip

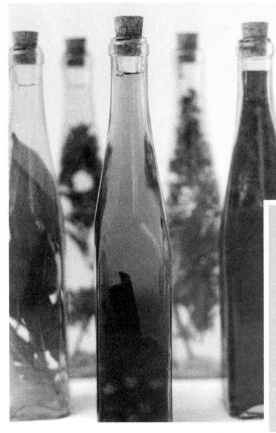

ingredients

Fat Free Balsamic Drizzle

2	cups balsamic vinegar
1/4	cup sugar in the raw
1	teaspoon fresh minced garlic
2	tablespoons fresh, finely minced basil
1	teaspoon dried Italian herb blend

Salt and pepper to taste

directions

■ Place vinegar and sugar in a non-reactive saucepan over medium heat and stir until sugar dissolves. Adjust heat to bring contents to a slow boil. Continue to boil slowly until mixture has reduced by one half. It should measure about 1 cup. Place in heatproof glass or ceramic container and cool. Stir in garlic and herbs. Season with salt and pepper. Serve over salad or anything grilled! Keeps 1 week tightly covered in the refrigerator.

Makes a little over 1 cup, serving 8 to 12.

ingredients

Quick Garlic Pickles

12	pickling cucumbers, washed
12	cloves, peeled fresh garlic
2	teaspoons dried dill weed
$1/2$	cup cider vinegar
$1^{1}/2$	cups water
1	tablespoon salt or to taste

Coarsely cracked pepper to taste

directions

- Slice the cucumbers into thick slices. Slice the garlic cloves into very thin slices. Place in a bowl or crock. Mix the dill with the vinegar, water and salt and pour over the cucumber garlic mixture. Sprinkle with cracked pepper to taste. Cover and refrigerate 48 hours. Enjoy!

Refrigerator Essentials

ingredients

Garlic Parmesan Vinaigrette

1	tablespoon fresh minced garlic
	Juice from 2 fresh lemons
2	teaspoons Worcestershire sauce
	cracked pepper to taste
1	cup grated parmesan cheese
	About $1/2$ cup extra virgin olive oil

directions

- Place the garlic, lemon juice, Worcestershire sauce, pepper and cheese into the bowl of a food processor fitted with a steel blade or blender. Process, while slowly adding the oil in a stream until the mixture emulsifies into a mayonnaise-like texture.

Makes about 1 cup.

directions

The last can of garbanzo beans can quickly be turned into hummus, served with chips or pita triangles.

■ In a food processor fitted with a steel blade process the beans, garlic, lemon juice, parsley and sesame oil until ground and smooth. Slowly add the olive oil in a stream until the hummus is smooth and creamy. Season with salt and pepper to taste.

Makes about 4 cups serving 6 to 8.

ingredients

Hummus Among-Us

1   15 ounce can garbanzo
     beans, drained
2   cloves garlic
Juice from 2 fresh lemons
1/4 cup fresh parsley
1   teaspoon sesame oil
1/4 cup extra virgin olive oil
Salt and pepper to taste

ingredients

Red Hot Applesauce

8 to 10 apples, cored and sliced
1/8 cup "Red Hot" cinnamon
     candies
Zest from 1 lemon
Juice from 1 lemon

directions

■ Place all ingredients in a heavy saucepan or Dutch oven over medium heat and simmer, stirring frequently, until the apples are tender and the candies have melted. Continue to simmer until apples are soft. Remove from heat and cool until warm. Run the mixture through a food mill to remove skin (Alternatively, you may remove the skins before cooking and puree the mixture.)

Makes about 6 cups of applesauce.

Refrigerator Essentials from the Market

Dairy

Skim Milk

Skim Chocolate Milk

No-Fat Natural Cottage Cheese

Assorted Flavors of nonfat Natural Yogurt

Plain nonfat Natural Yogurt

Assorted Low Fat Natural Cheeses

Low or nonfat Natural Cream Cheese

Organic Eggs or Natural Egg Substitute

Produce

Ready to eat Celery (organic if possible)

Ready to eat Carrots (organic if possible)

Organic Lemons

Bags of Organic Greens

Cut Up Watermelon Chunks

Organic Apples

Organic Seedless Oranges

Organic Sprouts

Beverages

Natural Flavors of Calorie Free Sparkling Waters

Water

Organic Unsweetened Juices

Condiments

Natural Mustards

Natural Catsup

Low or nonfat Natural Mayonnaise

Low or nonfat Natural Salad Dressing

Natural Sweet Pickle Relish

Misc.

Natural Whole Grain Tortillas

Shaved Smoked Preservative Free Turkey

Freezer

Natural Frozen Low or NonFat Yogurt

Natural Frozen Unsweetened All Fruit/Juice Bars

Whole Grain Natural Frozen Toaster Waffles

Natural Soy Bacon Substitute

Natural Soy Breakfast Sausage Links

Pantry Essentials from the Market

Baked Natural Pita Chips

Baked Natural Tortilla Chips

Natural Low Sodium nonfat Crackers/Flatbreads

Garbanzo Beans in the can

Natural Black Beans in the can

Natural nonfat Refried Beans in the can

Natural Corn Kernels in the can

Natural Salsa in the Jar

Dolphin Safe Albacore Tuna packed in Water

Maple Syrup

Organic Peanut Butter

All Fruit no sugar Jams and Jellies

Organic Unbleached Flour

Natural Baking Powder

Organic Brown Sugar

Organic Cane Sugar

Natural Pudding Mix you can make with Skim Milk

Extra Virgin Olive Oil

Canola Oil

Sesame Oil

Balsamic Vinegar

Seasoned Rice Vinegar

Cider Vinegar

Natural Vanilla Extract

Dried Italian Herb Blend

Dried Basil

Ground Cumin

Chili Powder

Curry Powder

Sea Salt

Ground Pepper

Toasted Sesame Seeds

Natural Spinach Pasta

Natural Red Pasta Sauces

Natural Low Fat Granolas

Low or No Sugar Breakfast Cereals

Natural Quick-Cook Oatmeal

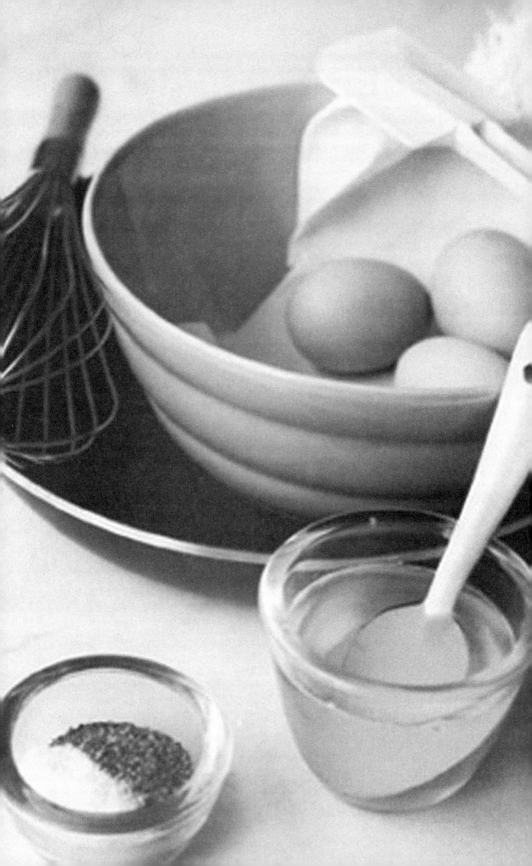

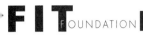
Breakfast

I travel a lot and like to stay at the same hotel in many places that I visit, as I am a creature of habit. I often get to know the front desk and housekeeping staff on a first name basis. In one hotel in particular, I have become friendly enough with several of the people who work there that we have had conversations about my weight loss.

One morning I came down to the lobby for my complimentary breakfast and one of my regulars flew out from behind the front desk. "I need your help!" she exclaimed. She lamented that as she aged her backside was getting wider and wider and, no matter what she did, no matter how many diets she tried, she absolutely could not lose weight and she felt she was spiraling out of control. How well I could relate to her!

The complimentary breakfast served at this hotel consisted of two sections. One side had waffles, sausage patties, gravy, cheesy eggs, pastry, bagels and donuts. The other side had fresh fruit, assorted cereals, granola and every flavor of low fat natural yogurt you could imagine.

I asked my expanding friend if she had enjoyed breakfast yet as I felt breakfast was a good place to start with the choices she was going to make for the rest of the day. "Why yes," she said, and continued, "I just had a small breakfast: two or three sausage patties covered with just a bit of gravy!"

Oh, dear sister, where do I begin? I was surprised that anyone who was so obsessed with wanting to lose weight would have made those choices. Surely the right choices were obvious, at least to me. But she then shared with me that she was used to eating the sausages and

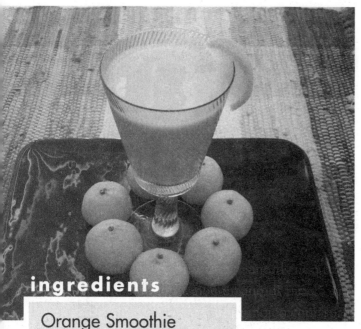

ingredients

Orange Smoothie

8 ounces orange yogurt
1 scoop orange sherbert
1 seedless orange, peeled
   and divided into sections

directions

■ Place the ingredients in blender and puree until smooth. Pour into a tall glass and serve immediately.

Serves 1

gravy with eggs and waffles along with donuts and coffee with cream. She felt she was cutting back and in fact, she was.

I then chose to explain to her that she could make some other choices that would not only lead to less calorie intake but would fill her up more and be a more healthy way for her to begin her day. I had her come with me to the breakfast buffet and showed her how I mixed cereal and yogurt in a bowl and then topped it with fresh fruit. I poured coffee over ice and added skim milk for a quick iced latte. I even explained that she could add some chocolate syrup to the latte and enjoy an iced mocha latte which would not only be deliciously satisfying and fat free but would kill her craving for sweets.

Start your day in a powerful, healthy way!

Breakfast

ingredients

Very Berry Breakfast Parfaits

16 ounces low fat yogurt of
    choice
2   cups raspberries or
    blueberries or both
2   cups granola of choice
1/2 cup unsweetened shredded
    coconut
1/2 yogurt covered raisins
4   perfect strawberries

directions

- In a tall, clear, plastic glass, alternate layers of the yogurt, berries and granola as desired. Top with coconut and raisins as desired. Place a perfect strawberry on top.

Makes 4 parfaits!

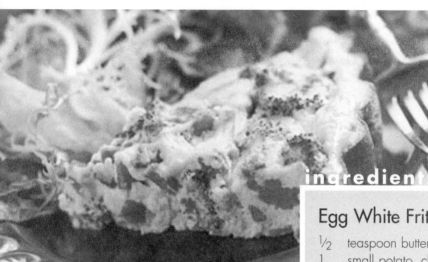

ingredients

Egg White Frittata

$1/2$ teaspoon butter
1   small potato, chopped
$1/4$ cup chopped scallions
$1/4$ cup chopped asparagus
1   red bell pepper, seeded
     and chopped
$1/8$ cup fresh chopped parsley
Salt and pepper to taste
8   egg whites
1   tablespoon grated
     parmesan cheese

directions

*This will work best in a heavy bottomed quality non-stick ovenproof pan. Egg whites are **very** sticky and if you don't have a non-stick pan, you may want to double the butter or oil.*

■ Heat the butter or oil in a heavy, non-stick 8 to 10 inch ovenproof saute pan over medium high heat and coat the pan with the fat. Sauté the potato and scallions until they begin to turn golden and add the asparagus, bell pepper and parsley and sauté a few minutes more. Season with salt and pepper to taste. Whisk the egg whites until frothy and pour them into the pan over the vegetables. Sprinkle the cheese over the top and place in a pre-heated 450-degree oven and bake until golden brown on top and set, about 5-7 minutes. Cut in half or thirds and serve immediately.

Serves 2 or 3.

ingredients

Veggie Egg White Omelet

1/4	teaspoon butter
2	fresh chopped scallions
1/4	cup chopped red pepper
1/4	cup chopped broccoli or cauliflower
2 to 3	chopped basil leaves
4 to 6	egg whites
Salt and pepper to taste	

directions

- Heat a medium sized non-stick omelet or sauté pan over medium high heat and brush with butter. Sauté vegetables for about 2 minutes and stir in basil. Beat egg whites until slightly foamy and pour over vegetables. Sprinkle with salt and pepper to taste. Flip sides in to create burrito shaped omelet or fold in half for a half moon shape. Flip and brown on both sides.

Serves 1.

directions

- Mix together the pumpkin, flour, baking powder, cinnamon, clove, sugar and vanilla until smooth. Blend in the eggs. Heat a large, heavy non-stick skillet over medium-high heat and swirl around just enough butter to season the pan. Spoon the batter into 3-inch circles onto the hot skillet and reduce heat to medium, cooking the pancakes to brown on one side, about 2 or 3 minutes. Carefully turn the pancakes and brown on the other side for the same amount of time. Serve hot with maple syrup or blueberry jam.

Makes about 18 pancakes.

ingredients

Pumpkin Pancakes

1	cup pumpkin flesh purée, either canned or fresh
1 1/2	cups unbleached all purpose flour
1	teaspoon baking powder
1	teaspoon ground cinnamon
1/2	teaspoon ground clove
1	cup granulated sugar
1	teaspoon vanilla extract
2	eggs
Butter for frying	

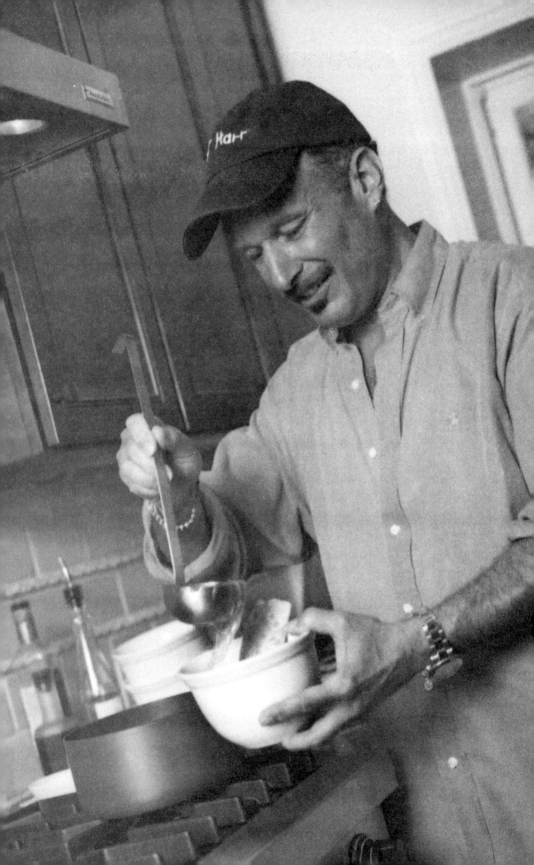

Soups

The discovery of being served a thick, creamy soup inside a hollowed out round loaf of bread was like going to the culinary moon for me. Who could be so brilliant as to make it easy to eat a high fat, high carb soup such as New England Clam Chowder and then the soggy loaf of bread as a chaser? I used to enjoy an order of fries or onion rings on the side! Now when I see that on a menu I just shake my head.

In fact, soups and stews can be a deliciously healthy and filling way to enjoy a meal. We do, however, have to choose a little wiser and the bread bowl is out. Instead, make or purchase a crispy flatbread or bread stick and serve these on the side. I also like to break up the flatbread and ladle the soup on top!

Hearty soups are very filling and satisfying. They are a great opportunity to combine protein with a dose of vegetables and grains while keeping them virtually fat free. What could be better after a hard day a school than a chunky bowl of soup?

FIT OUNDATION tip

71

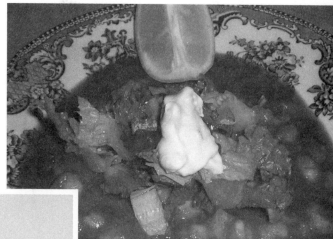

ingredients

Hominy Soup

2	tablespoons olive oil
1	onion, minced
4	cloves garlic, minced
45	ounces (3 cans) hominy, drained
3	cups tomato sauce

juice from 2 fresh limes

1	teaspoon mild chili powder
1	tablespoon ground cumin
2	cups vegetable or chicken stock

Garnishes:

Shredded lettuce
Fat free sour cream
Chopped avocado
Sliced jalapeños
Shredded cheddar cheese
Shredded cooked chicken
Wedges of lemon or lime

directions

This may be made a day or two in advance, cooled, covered, refrigerated and reheated before serving.

■ In a 3-quart or larger, heavy bottomed non corrosive saucepan or stock pot, heat the oil over medium high heat and in it saute the onion until golden. Stir in the garlic and saute another minute or two. Stir in the drained hominy, tomato sauce, lime juice, chili powder, cumin and stock. Stir to blend well. Reduce heat and bring to a simmer, stirring occasionally, for 10 to 15 minutes. Serve hot with garnishes of choice.

Serves 6 as an entree or 8 as a soup course.

ingredients

Southwestern Chicken Soup

1	tablespoon canola oil
1	large onion, chopped
4	carrots, chopped
4	stalks celery, chopped
2	Anaheim chiles, seeded and chopped
4	skinless, boneless chicken breasts, spilt
1	tablespoon salt
1 1/2	liters spring water
1	rutabaga
1	pound new potatoes
24	ounces tomato puree
1/2	cup fresh chopped cilantro leaf
1	teaspoon dried oregano
1/8	cup ground cumin
1	teaspoon paprika

Juice from 3 lemons
Avocado slices and fat free sour cream for garnish

directions

- In a large, heavy soup pot, heat the oil over medium high heat and stir in the onion, carrots, celery and chiles. Sauté until slightly golden. Place chicken breasts in pot on top of vegetables and cook for 2 minutes undisturbed. Sprinkle with salt and cover with water. When pot begins to boil, reduce heat to maintain low boil and cook until chicken is tender, about an hour. Remove chicken and strain stock through a cheese cloth and place stock back into pot. Chop the cooked onion, carrots, celery and chiles and set aside. Shred the chicken and set aside. Clean rutabaga and potatoes and cut them into small chunks and place in the pot with the stock. Simmer until rutabaga and potatoes are tender but still firm. Stir in tomato puree, cilantro, oregano, cumin, paprika and lemon juice. Simmer slowly for 20 minutes to allow flavors to merge. Add chopped onion, carrots, celery, chiles and shredded chicken. Bring soup back to a simmer. Serve in warm bowls and garnish with avocado and sour cream.

Serves 8.

Soups

ingredients

Sesame Egg Drop Soup with Chicken

12	cups chicken or vegetable stock
3	eggs, slightly beaten
1/4	cup soy sauce
2	tablespoons fresh minced ginger
1/2	cup sake or dry vermouth
2	cups diced cooked chicken
6	ounces fresh baby spinach, washed well
12	ounces fresh bean sprouts, rinsed

Chopped scallions and toasted sesame seeds for garnish

directions

■ Bring the stock to a slow simmer and, while whisking gently in a circular motion, pour in the egg in a slow stream which will create egg "flowers." Add the soy sauce, ginger and sake to the soup along with the chicken chunks. Bring back to a slow simmer. *Never boil!* Just before serving, add the spinach to the soup. Divide the sprouts among 8 bowls and ladle the soup over the sprouts. Garnish with scallions and sesame seeds.

Serves 8.

ingredients

Loaded Chunky Vegetable Soup

2	tablespoons extra virgin olive oil
2	medium onions, peeled and chopped
5	small gold potatoes, scrubbed and cut into small chunks
2	turnips, peeled and chunked
2	parsnips, peeled and chunked
1/2	cup extra dry vermouth
1/2	cup fresh chopped parsley
8	cups bottled water
1/2	cup chopped sorrel
3	cups chopped broccoli
1	teaspoon ground black pepper
1	tablespoon dried Italian herb blend
1	red pepper, seeded and chopped
4	stalks celery, chopped
2	cups sliced baby carrots
8	ounces oyster mushrooms or mushrooms of choice

Soups

directions

- In a large soup pot, heat the oil over medium high heat and in it sauté the onion until it begins to toast, about 7 minutes. Add the potato, turnip and parsnip to the pot, reduce heat to medium, and sauté another 4 minutes. Add vermouth to pot and then stir in parsley and half of the water. Reduce heat to simmer contents for 5 minutes. Add sorrel and broccoli to pot along with pepper and herbs to taste. Add the remaining water and bring back to a simmer. Add red pepper, celery, and carrots to pot and continue to simmer until cooked to your liking. 10 minutes before serving, add oyster mushrooms to pot. Season with salt and additional pepper as desired.

Serves 8.

ingredients

Beef Barley Soup

3	tablespoons olive oil
2 to 4	pounds beef soup bones, trimmed of fat
3	onions, minced
3	cloves garlic, minced
1/2	cup barley
8	cups water
1	teaspoon dried Italian herb blend
4	stalks celery, chopped
4	carrots diced
	Salt and pepper to taste
1/2	cup fresh chopped parsley

directions

■ In a stockpot or Dutch oven, heat the olive oil over high heat and in it, brown the soup bones, stirring constantly, for about 5 minutes. Stir in the onion and garlic and sauté another 2 minutes. Stir in the barley and sauté another couple of minutes and then stir in the water. Bring to a simmer and adjust heat to maintain a simmer. Cover loosely and simmer until barley is tender. If any foam collects on top, skim it off during this process. Remove the bones from the soup and remove the meat and marrow from the bones and chop. Place it back in the soup and discard the bones. Add the herbs, celery and carrots to the pot and simmer until the vegetables are tender. Season with salt and pepper. Keep warm until ready to serve and, just before serving, stir in the parsley. Serve with crusty bread and slices of aged cheddar for a delicious lunch or supper.

Serves 6.

ingredients

Black Bean Soup

2	tablespoons canola oil
2	minced onions
2	cloves fresh minced garlic
2	carrots, diced
4	stalks celery, diced
1/2	cup fresh chopped cilantro
3	tablespoons mild chili powder
3	tablespoons ground cumin
12	ounces dried black beans, rinsed and picked over
8	cups water

directions

Leftovers of this tasty and fill-ing soup can be heated and poured over baked tortilla chips and topped with low fat ched-dar for a terrific snack or meal.

Garnishes: sour cream, shredded cheddar cheese, minced jalapeños, chopped red onion, and shred-ded lettuce

■ Place the oil in large heavy soup pot or Dutch oven over medium-high heat and sauté the onion, garlic, carrots and celery until toasted. Stir in the cilantro, chili powder, cumin, beans and water to the pot. Mix well and cover loosely. Adjust heat to simmer and stirring frequently, cook for 3 or 4 hours, until beans are tender. Serve with garnish-es. Serves 6 to 8 for lunch or up to 12 as a first course. Sliced grilled chicken may be arranged on top of the soup for a full meal in 1 bowl!

Serves 6-8.

Soups

ingredients

Broccoli Cheddar Soup

2   tablespoons butter
1   onion, minced
4   cups chopped broccoli
1   tablespoon Italian herb blend
2   tablespoons unbleached all
      purpose flour
12   ounces light beer
2   cups low fat shredded cheddar
      cheese
4   cups skim milk
Salt and pepper to taste

directions

- In a large heavy Dutch oven or saucepan over medium high heat, melt the butter and stir in the onion, broccoli and herbs. Sauté, stirring frequently, until the onion is golden and the broccoli is tender. Stir in the flour. Cook two minutes more and slowly stir in the beer and cook until the mixture thickens and bubbles and the alcohol burns off, about 3 minutes. Stir in cheese and add about 1/4 of the milk. Stir constantly until cheese melts and slowly add the balance of the milk while continuing to stir. Simmer gently for a moment and season with salt and pepper to taste. Serve immediately. For a one-dish supper, add sliced warm grilled chicken to soup and serve with crisp herbed flatbread.

Serves 4 to 6

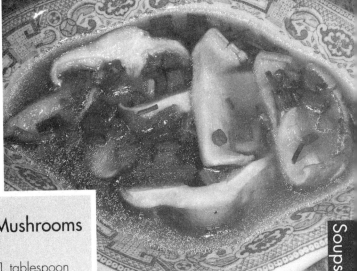

Soups

ingredients

Miso Soup with Mushrooms

6	cups water
1/3	cup dark miso or 1 tablespoon per serving
2	tablespoons freshly minced ginger
8	ounces extra firm tofu cut into small cubes
16	ounces fresh white mushrooms, trimmed, rinsed and sliced
1	bunch scallions, trimmed and chopped
	toasted sesame seeds to taste
2	cups bean sprouts

directions

■ Bring the water to a simmer. Place the miso in a heatproof cup and stir in enough hot water to make a thin paste. Stir the miso paste and ginger into the water. Keep hot but not boiling. A few minutes before serving, add tofu to soup along with mushrooms, scallions and sesame seeds and cook until tofu is hot and mushrooms are tender. Place bean sprouts in bottom of presentation bowl(s) and ladle soup over sprouts. Serve with sesame hot oil if desired.

Serves 4 to 6.

ingredients

Beef Stew

3 to 4 pounds lean chuck cut into small cubes
3 tablespoons canola oil
2 onions, diced
1 celery heart, cut into small chunks
3 cloves garlic, sliced thinly
2 tablespoons soy sauce
2 cups red wine
4 cups beef stock or bouillon
1 tablespoon dried Italian herb blend
1 teaspoon ground pepper
1 cup tomato sauce
2 or 3 potatoes, scrubbed and cut into small chunks
2 cups baby carrots, cut in half
2/3 cup seasoned bread crumbs
1 cup frozen peas

directions

■ Rinse the beef and pat dry with paper towels. In a heavy Dutch oven over medium high heat, heat the oil and brown the beef in 3 or 4 batches. Remove the beef from the pan. In the same pan, sauté the onion for about 5 minutes and add the celery and garlic to the pan. Sauté another two minutes and return the beef to the pan. Add the soy sauce and red wine to the pan and reduce heat to medium. Simmer for 5 minutes and add the stock to the pan. Stir in the herbs and pepper. Cover loosely and reduce heat to medium low.

Simmer contents of pan gently for about 2 hours or until beef is very tender. Add tomato sauce and potatoes to pan. Simmer another 10 minutes and stir in carrots. Simmer another 10 minutes and stir in breadcrumbs until juice is as thick as desired. Stir in the peas and cook just until peas are hot. Serve immediately or cool, cover and refrigerate over night. Reheat before serving. **Note:** To stretch this recipe, serve the stew over cooked rice or slices of crusty bread. *Serves 6.*

ingredients

Sweet and Sour Cabbage Stew

3   tablespoons vegetable oil
2   pounds extra lean ground beef
1   medium white onion, diced
2   cloves garlic, minced
2   pounds shredded white cabbage (2 heads)
1   cup extra dry vermouth
16   ounces tomato sauce
2   cups beef stock
Juice from 2 fresh lemons
1/3 cup light brown sugar
1/4 cup maple syrup
Salt and pepper to taste
1/4 cup seasoned bread crumbs

directions

- In a large soup pot or Dutch oven over medium high heat, add the oil and in it sauté the beef while scrambling until brown. Add onion and garlic and sauté another 5 minutes. Reduce the heat to medium and place the shredded cabbage in the pot over the beef mixture. Drizzle the vermouth over the cabbage and cover loosely either with a lid or with foil. Reduce heat to medium low. When cabbage has wilted and is beginning to become tender, stir to combine with the beef. Stir in the tomato sauce and the beef stock and bring to a simmer. Season with the lemon juice, brown sugar and maple syrup to taste. Season again with salt and pepper to taste. Simmer for 90 minutes. Stir in bread crumbs and simmer until thick. Serve immediately or cool, cover and refrigerate over night. Reheat before serving.

Serves 6 to 8.

Soups

ingredients

Turkey Chili

2	tablespoons olive oil
2	chopped white onions
3	tablespoons fresh minced garlic
3 or 4	chopped seeded mild green chiles
2	teaspoons salt
60	ounces crushed tomatoes or tomato puree
3	tablespoons ground cumin or to taste
2	tablespoons mild chili powder or to taste
2	tablespoons paprika
2	tablespoons brown sugar or Sugar In The Raw
2 or 3	cans pinto beans, drained
3 or 4	cups leftover turkey, cut into chunks

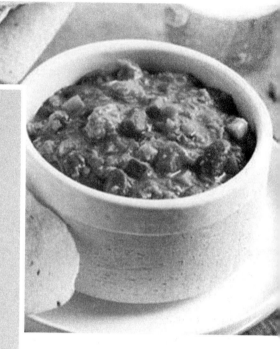

directions

Grated cheddar cheese, sour cream, chopped onion and jalapeño slices for garnish.

- Heat oil in large pot over medium high heat and stir in onion and garlic. Sauté for 5 minutes. Add chiles and salt and sauté 1 minute more. Stir in tomatoes and season with cumin, chili powder, paprika and sugar. Simmer 2 hours and re-season to taste. Stir in beans and turkey and cook until hot. Serve or cover, refrigerate and serve the next day (it is really better if it sits overnight). Heat and serve.

Serves 10 to 12.

ingredients

Chicken in a Pot

1	stewing chicken
2	carrots
4	stalks celery
1	onion
2	cloves garlic
1	bay leaf
2	sage leaves
1	small bunch fresh parsley

Salt and pepper to taste
2 or 3 cups cooked noodles or rice

directions

■ Rinse the chicken, trim off any fat and remove any liver or giblets. Place the chicken (and neck if there is one) in a slow cooker or stew pot and cover with water. Cut the carrots and celery into chunks and add to the water. Peel the onion and garlic and place in the pot with the chicken along with the bay and sage leaves. Rinse the parsley and tie in a bunch with kitchen twine and place in the water. Cover the cooker or pot and place over low heat and bring to a simmer. Simmer very gently and slowly until chicken is cooked and tender, skimming off any foam that gathers during the process. The simmering process could take 3 to 5 hours for a good, tender chicken to result. When done, remove everything from the broth and strain the broth back into a pot. Chop the cooked carrots, celery and onion and put back in the pot. Taste the broth and season with salt and pepper to taste. Remove the meat from the chicken bones, cut into bite sized pieces and place in the broth. Bring back to a simmer and, just before serving, add cooked noodles or rice to the pot.

Serves 6 to 8.

Soups

ingredients

Jesse James Soup

1	tablespoon canola oil
1	large onion, chopped
2	Anaheim chiles, seeded and chopped
4	skinless, boneless chicken breasts, split
1	tablespoon salt
1½	liters spring water
1	rutabaga
1	pound new potatoes
24	ounces tomato puree
½	cup chopped cilantro leaf
1	teaspoon dried oregano
⅛	cup ground cumin
1	teaspoon paprika
Juice from 3 lemons	

directions

Avocados, sour cream and sourdough croutons for garnish

■ In a large, heavy soup pot heat the oil over medium high heat and stir in the onions and chiles. Sauté until slightly golden. Place chicken breasts in pot on top of vegetables and cook for 2 minutes undisturbed. Sprinkle with salt and cover with water. When pot begins to boil, reduce heat to maintain low boil and cook until chicken is tender, about an hour. Remove chicken and strain stock through a cheese cloth and place back into pot. Clean rutabaga and potatoes and cut them into small chunks. Place in stock and simmer until tender but still firm. Stir in tomato puree, cilantro, oregano, cumin, paprika and lemon juice. Simmer slowly for 20 minutes to allow flavors to merge. Serve in warm bowls and garnish with avocado, sour cream and sourdough croutons.

Serves 6.

ingredients

Tofu Soup Pot

12	cups chicken or vegetable stock
3	eggs, slightly beaten
1/4	cup soy sauce
2	tablespoons fresh minced ginger
1/2	cup sake
12	ounces extra firm tofu, drained and cut into small squares
6	ounces fresh oyster mushrooms (optional)
6	ounces fresh baby spinach, washed well
12	ounces fresh bean sprouts, rinsed

directions

Chopped scallions and toasted sesame seeds for garnish

■ In a large soup pot, bring the stock to a slow simmer and, while whisking gently in a circular motion, pour in the egg in a slow stream, which will create egg "flowers." Add the soy sauce, ginger and sake to the soup along with the tofu. Bring back to a slow simmer. *Never boil!* Rinse and drain the mushrooms and trim off any tough stems. Add to the soup and cook for about 7 minutes. Just before serving, add the spinach to the soup. Divide the sprouts among 8 bowls and ladle the soup over the sprouts. Garnish with scallions and sesame seeds.

Serves 8.

Soups

ingredients

Hot & Sour Soup

2	ounces dried black mushrooms
1/2	cup dry sherry
2	tablespoons cornstarch
1	tablespoon soy sauce
7 to 8	cups chicken or vegetable stock
3	tablespoons catsup
1	teaspoon seasoned rice vinegar
2	eggs, beaten well
2	cups cooked white meat chicken, shredded
1	extra firm tofu cake, about 12 ounces, cut into cubes
1/2	cup scallion greens, chopped hot chili sesame oil to taste (available at Oriental markets and most supermarkets in the Asian dept.)

directions

■ Soak the mushrooms in the sherry until tender. Chop mushrooms. Stir enough of the remaining sherry into the cornstarch to form a smooth paste and then mix in the rest of the sherry and the soy sauce into the cornstarch mixture. Heat the stock until simmering and add the catsup, vinegar and soaked mushrooms. Stir rapidly while pouring the egg into the stock in a stream. Stir in cornstarch mixture and cook until soup thickens. Reduce heat and stir in chicken, tofu cubes and scallions. Stir in a few drops of hot chili sesame oil to taste.

Serves 6 to 8.

directions

■ Heat stock to a simmer. Lightly beat the eggs and, while stirring soup briskly, pour eggs in a slow stream. They will become feathery "flowers." Mix the cornstarch with the water and stir into the soup with catsup. Adjust heat to keep hot but not simmering. Serve with a sprinkle of scallions and sesame seeds. Season with soy sauce and hot oil to taste.

Serves 4.

ingredients

Egg Flower Soup

6	cups chicken or vegetable broth
3	eggs
1	tablespoon cornstarch
2	tablespoons water
2	tablespoons catsup
1/2	cup fresh chopped scallions
1/4	cup toasted sesame seeds
	Soy sauce & hot oil to taste

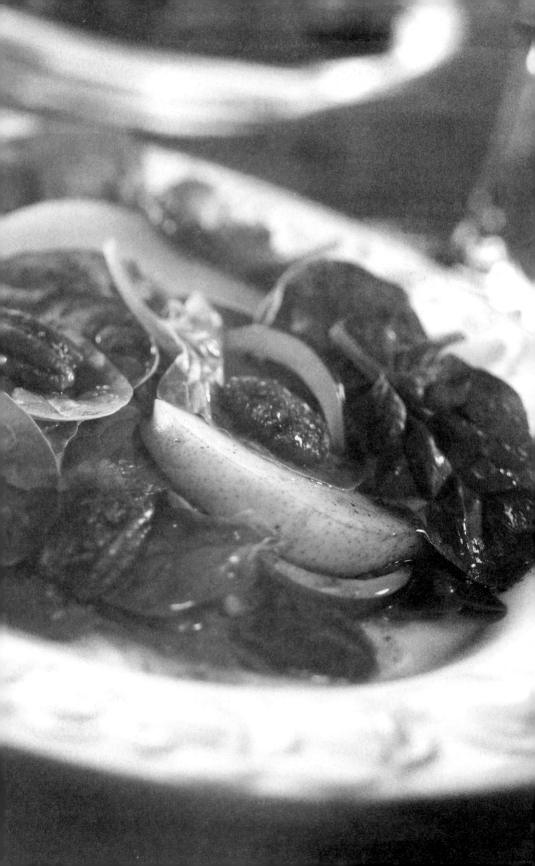

Salads that can be meals

I have always had a love affair with lettuce. It is a vegetable that is virtually calorie free, filling and satisfying. Scientist even claim it makes you sleep better when you eat lettuce and lettuce was once considered an aphrodisiac! It is readily available in many varieties (over 200) at grocery stores, green grocers, farmers markets, restaurants and cafeterias. It has been cultivated for thousands of years and is also easy and fun to grow yourself. Put some colorful varieties in window boxes or containers around the house. Harvest it for a quick meal! Lettuce is culinary ubiquity! How great that it also happens to be good for you. Load on lettuce and make it a meal. It is impossible to eat too much.

The ready washed bags of organic salad greens are the Fit Foundation version of fast food. Open a bag, add some low or nonfat dressing and perhaps some leftover grilled meat and you have a healthy delicious meal!

FIT Foundation tip

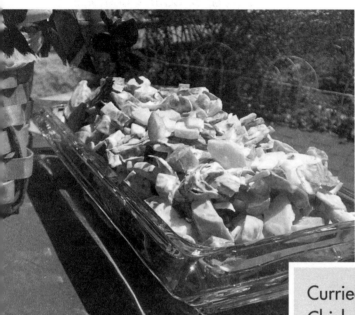

ingredients

Curried Grilled Chicken Salad

1 1/3 cups low or nonfat mayonnaise or plain yogurt

1/2 cup nonfat lemon yogurt

1 teaspoon or to taste curry powder or curry blend

2 to 3 cups grilled chicken chunks

2/3 cup diced celery

1 cup chopped almonds

2/3 cup golden raisins

3 chopped hard-boiled eggs

directions

■ In a mixing bowl, stir together the mayonnaise, yogurt and curry until blended. Stir in remaining ingredients to mix well. Cover and refrigerate for a few hours before serving. Stuff into hollowed red bell peppers for serving, if desired.

Serves 4.

ingredients

Sweet & Sour Cucumbers

2	cucumbers
2	small purple onions
1	cup fresh chopped parsley
2/3	cup red wine vinegar
1 1/3	cups water
1	teaspoon dried Italian herb blend
1/8	cup sugar
	Salt and pepper to taste

directions

■ Slice the cucumbers thinly and place in a bowl. Thinly slice the onions and separate into rings and place in the bowl with the cucumbers. Add the parsley to the bowl. Mix the vinegar, water, herbs and sugar together and season with salt and pepper to taste. Pour the dressing over the cucumbers, onions and parsley and toss. Cover with plastic wrap and refrigerate, tossing occasionally, for 24 hours.

Serves 8 as a salad or side dish.

ingredients

Yellow Tomato, Mint and Lime Salsa

4	firm yellow tomatoes, seeded and chopped
1	red pepper, trimmed and chopped
1	tablespoon extra virgin olive oil
2	tablespoons fresh mint leaf, minced
6	scallions, chopped
	Juice from 2 fresh limes
	Salt and pepper to taste

directions

■ Toss all ingredients gently to combine and season with salt and pepper to taste.

Makes about 2 cups.

Salads

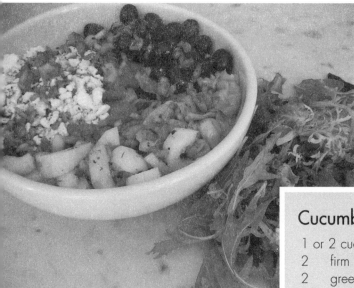

ingredients

Cucumber Greek Salad

1 or 2 cucumbers
2   firm but ripe tomatoes
2   green bell peppers
1   cup fresh rinsed basil
    leaves
8 to 10 ounces feta cheese
½ cup pitted kalamata olives,
    drained
The juice from 2 fresh lemons
Extra virgin olive oil to taste

directions

■ Peel and seed the cucumber and cut into chunks. Seed the tomatoes and cut them into chunks, too. Slice the peppers thinly. Arrange the vegetables on a serving platter and place the basil leaves attractively around the edge of the vegetables. Crumble the cheese over the top of the vegetables and dot the olives over the cheese. Drizzle the lemon juice over the top and then drizzle the olive oil over that. Serve immediately. Cooked and chilled shrimp may be added for a delicious entrée salad.

Serves 4.

ingredients

Cucumber Salad

2	cucumbers
1	bunch scallions
2	tablespoons snipped fresh dill
1	cup plain non-fat yogurt
1	teaspoon white wine vinegar

Salt and pepper to taste

directions

■ Peel, seed and slice the cucumbers. Toss with the scallions. Mix the dill into the yogurt with the vinegar. Combine the yogurt mixture with the cucumbers and scallions to coat. Season with salt and pepper. Serve with thin slices of smoked salmon for an elegant summer's day lunch.

Serves 6 to 8 as a salad.

ingredients

Tofu Mayonnaise

1	12 to 16 ounce block soft, silken tofu
4	tablespoons white wine vinegar

Juice from 1 fresh lemon
2/3 cup extra virgin olive oil
Salt and white pepper to taste

directions

■ In a food processor fitted with a steel blade, process the tofu until smooth. Add the vinegar to the bowl and pulse to combine. Scrape the sides of the bowl. Turn on the machine and add the lemon, then add the oil in a slow stream and process until thick and rich looking. Season with salt and pepper. Cover and refrigerate up to 10 days.

Makes about 2 cups.

Salads

ingredients

Sweet Potato Lentil Salad

8	ounces dried lentils
12	cups water
1 or 2	sweet potatoes
1	bunch scallions
1	red bell pepper
1/2	cup extra virgin olive oil
1	teaspoon dried Italian herbs
1	teaspoon maple syrup
2	teaspoons seasoned rice vinegar (as for sushi)

Salt and pepper to taste

directions

■ Simmer the lentils in half of the water until firmly tender but not mushy, about 25 to 30 minutes. Drain in a colander and rinse in cold water to stop the cooking process. Peel and slice the sweet potato into small, 1/2 inch thick pieces and simmer in the other half of the water until firmly tender but not mushy, about 20 minutes. Drain and run under cold water. Trim, chop and rinse the scallions and bell pepper. Place the lentils, sweet potato, scallions and pepper in a mixing bowl that will accommodate tossing. In another smaller spouted bowl, whisk together the oil, herbs and syrup. Whisk in the vinegar. (Please be certain it is *seasoned* rice vinegar as plain rice vinegar is extremely tart.) Season with salt and pepper to taste and pour the dressing over the vegetables and toss well to combine. Serve immediately or cover and refrigerate up to 48 hours before serving. Toss well prior to serving. *Serves 6.*

ingredients

Rosemary Roasted Potato Salad

3 or 4 pounds potatoes, scrubbed
    and cut into small chunks
2   onions, chopped
2   red bell peppers, trimmed and
    chopped
1/2 cup olive oil
Several sprigs fresh rosemary,
    stems discarded
1   tablespoon seasoned salt
2   cups balsamic vinegar
1/2 cup granulated sugar
1   teaspoon dried Italian herbs
Salt to taste
Fresh cracked pepper to taste

directions

■ Toss the potatoes, onions and peppers with the olive oil and place in a single layer on a baking sheet. Sprinkle the rosemary leaves over the vegetables and then sprinkle with seasoned salt to taste. Roast the potatoes in a preheated 325-degree oven until crisp on the outside and tender but firm on the inside, about 35 to 45 minutes. Remove to a rack to cool and scrape the contents of the baking pan into a mixing bowl. While the potatoes are roasting, heat the vinegar and sugar in a small non-reactive pan and simmer until reduced by half in volume. Remove from heat and stir in the dried herbs and salt to taste. Cool to room temperature and pour over the vegetables in the mixing bowl. Toss well to mix. Top with fresh cracked pepper to taste.

Serves 6 to 8.

Salads

directions

- Using a fork, mix together the garlic, herbs, pepper, paprika, salt, vinegar and lemon juice. Whisk in the oil in a slow stream and add crushed red pepper to taste.

Makes about 1 cup.

ingredients

Zesty Italian Dressing

1	tablespoon fresh minced garlic
1	teaspoon Italian herb blend
$1/2$	teaspoon ground pepper
$1/2$	teaspoon sweet paprika
$1/2$	teaspoon salt
2	tablespoons red wine vinegar

Juice from 1 lemon
$2/3$ cup extra virgin olive oil
Crushed red pepper to taste

ingredients

Rosemary Balsamic Drizzle

2	cups balsamic vinegar
$1/2$	cup granulated sugar
1	teaspoon fresh minced garlic
2	tablespoons finely minced fresh basil

one or two sprigs of fresh rosemary
salt and pepper to taste

directions

- Place vinegar and sugar in a non-reactive saucepan over medium heat and stir until sugar dissolves. Adjust heat to bring contents to a slow boil.

Continue to boil slowly until mixture has reduced by one half. It should measure about 1 cup. Place in heatproof glass or ceramic container and cool. Stir in garlic and the sprig(s) of fresh rosemary. Remove and discard the rosemary at the end of simmering. Season with salt and pepper. Serve over salad or anything grilled! Keeps for 1 week tightly covered in the refrigerator.

Makes a little over 1 cup, serving 8 to 12.

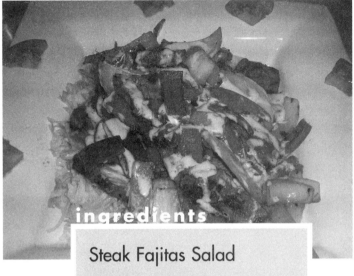

directions

Serve this over shredded lettuce with salsa, fresh minced jalapeños, sliced avocado and reduced-fat sour cream. Tortillas are optional.

■ Wrap the steaks in a single layer in plastic wrap and place them in a plastic bag and then freeze for 2 hours. Slice the meat across the grain into thin slices. Set aside. Heat one tablespoon of the oil in a large, heavy saute pan over high heat and stir fry the onions, garlic and bell peppers, about 20 minutes and add the tomato. Sauté for 30 seconds and remove from the pan to a heat-proof dish. Replace the pan to the heat and add the remaining tablespoon of vegetable oil to the pan. Brown the meat in the oil and add the vegetables back to the pan. Season with the soy sauce, cumin and chili powder to taste. Squeeze the limes over the pan and serve hot and sizzling.

Serves 4 to 6.

ingredients

Steak Fajitas Salad

2 or 3	lean strip steaks
2	tablespoons vegetable oil
2	medium sweet onions, sliced thinly
1	tablespoon fresh minced garlic
1	red Bell pepper, seeded and sliced into strips
1	green Bell pepper, seeded and sliced into strips
2	tomatoes, seeded and sliced into strips
1	teaspoon soy sauce
1	tablespoon ground cumin
1 or 2	teaspoons ground mild chili powder
3	fresh limes, cut in half

Salads

97

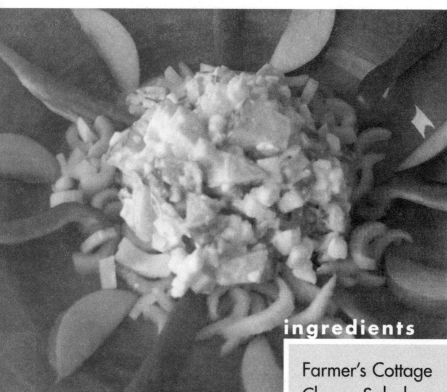

ingredients

directions

■ Mix all ingredients together and serve. This can be made ahead, 24 hours, covered and refrigerated and stirred again just before serving.

Serves 4 to 6.

Farmer's Cottage Cheese Salad

3   cups nonfat creamy
     small curd cottage cheese
1   bunch scallions, trimmed
     and chopped
1   bell pepper, seeded and
     chopped
1/4 cup chopped fresh parsley
6 to 8 radishes, trimmed and
     chopped
1   tablespoon fresh minced
     basil
Cracked fresh pepper to taste

ingredients

Creamy Cucumber Salad

2 or 3 English or "burp-less' cucumbers
2 red bell peppers, seeded and chunked
1 red onion
1 tablespoon red wine vinegar
2 cups low fat sour cream
1 teaspoon dried oregano
1 teaspoon raw cane sugar
Salt and pepper to taste

directions

■ Split the cucumbers down the middle and run a spoon down the center to remove the seeds and discard. Slice the cucumbers into thin slices and place the slices in a glass or ceramic mixing bowl with the chunks of bell pepper. Mince the onion and place with the cucumber. Mix the vinegar into the sour cream and blend in the oregano, sugar and salt and pepper to taste. Pour over the cucumber, peppers and minced onion and toss to coat. Cover and refrigerate up to 24 hours before serving. Mix together well before serving.

Serves 8 to 12.

Salads

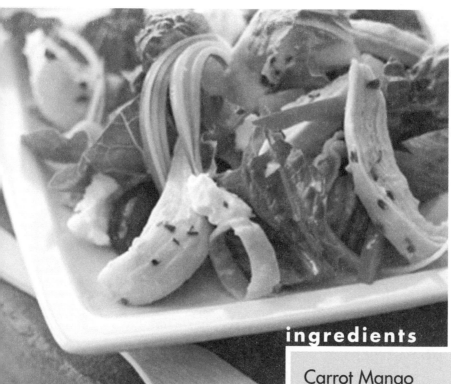

ingredients

Carrot Mango Chicken Salad

1   cup mango - chopped into
     small chunks
¹/₄ cup fresh chopped cilantro
     leaves
juice from 3 medium limes
¹/₄ cup minced white onion
1¹/₂ cups shredded carrots
1   tablespoon sugar
salt and pepper to taste
organic mixed baby greens
4   chilled grilled chicken
     breasts, sliced

directions

- Combine all ingredients except the greens and chicken in a bowl. Let sit for 20 minutes or so for flavors to combine. Serve on a bed of greens with the chicken on top.

Serves 8.

ingredients

Roasted White Corn and Multi Bean Salad

4	ears fresh white corn, cleaned
1	can organic prepared white beans, drained
1	can organic prepared black beans, drained
1	can organic prepared pinto beans, drained
1	can organic prepared red kidney beans, drained
1/2	cup fresh minced cilantro
	juice from 4 limes
1	tablespoon fresh ground sweet chili powder
2	tablespoons fresh ground cumin

salt to taste

directions

- In a non-stick skillet that will accommodate the corn, toast the corn over medium high heat for about 3 minutes per side, turning quarter turns, until kernels begin to brown. Cool and remove kernels from cob with a sharp knife or corn cobber. Rinse and drain beans and toss with corn, cilantro, lime juice, chili powder, and cumin. Salt to taste.

Salads

ingredients

Marinated Shrimp & Roasted Peppers

4	firm red bell peppers
1	sweet onion
1/4	cup safflower oil
2	tablespoons fresh minced garlic
1/8	cup soy sauce
1/4	cup extra virgin olive oil
1/4	cup red wine vinegar
1	teaspoon granulated sugar
1/4	cup fresh chopped basil
1	tablespoon minced oregano leaf

a dash or two of hot sauce or cayenne pepper if desired

salt and pepper to taste

1 pound large cooked, cleaned cocktail shrimp, no tails

directions

■ Cut peppers in half, clean and quarter. Slice onion. Mix safflower oil, 1 tablespoon of the garlic and soy sauce together. Drizzle over onions and peppers. Marinate 30 minutes. Grill peppers and onion slices over medium hot coals until skins begin to blister on peppers and onions are tender. Remove from grill. Slice into chunks. Mix together olive oil, the other tablespoon of garlic, vinegar, sugar, basil, oregano, hot sauce, salt and pepper. Toss peppers and onions with shrimp. Pour olive oil/ vinegar mixture over and toss again. Serves 6-8 as an appetizer. Can be made 24 hours in advance. Remove from refrigerator 30 minutes before serving.

Serves 6-8 as an appetizer.

ingredients

Tuna in Red

16	ounces fancy albacore white meat tuna in spring water
1	cup bottled chili sauce
1	teaspoon mild chili powder
$1/8$	cup prepared horseradish
1	teaspoon cracked pepper
1	teaspoon fresh lemon juice
1	cup chunked pickled cauli flower, drained
1	cup sliced, pitted green olives, drained
$1/2$	cup chunked, seeded sweet red pepper
1	cup chopped celery
$1/2$	cup chopped onion

directions

■ Cut peppers in half, clean and Mix together tuna, chili sauce, chili powder, horseradish, cracked pepper and lemon juice with a fork to break up chunks of tuna. Stir in remaining ingredients. Cover and refrigerate until serving.

Serves 6-8 over greens as an entree salad.

directions

■ Whisk together the mayonnaise, vinegar and sour cream. Season with salt, pepper and sugar. Mix with cabbage, carrots and scallions and toss to coat well. Cover and refrigerate 2 hours or overnight.

Serves 8 to 10.

ingredients

Cole Slaw

1	cup no or low fat mayonnaise
$1/4$	cup red wine vinegar
$1/3$	cup nonfat sour cream
Salt and pepper to taste	
2	tablespoons sugar
6	cups finely shredded white cabbage
1	cup shredded carrots
1	cup fresh chopped scallion greens

Salads

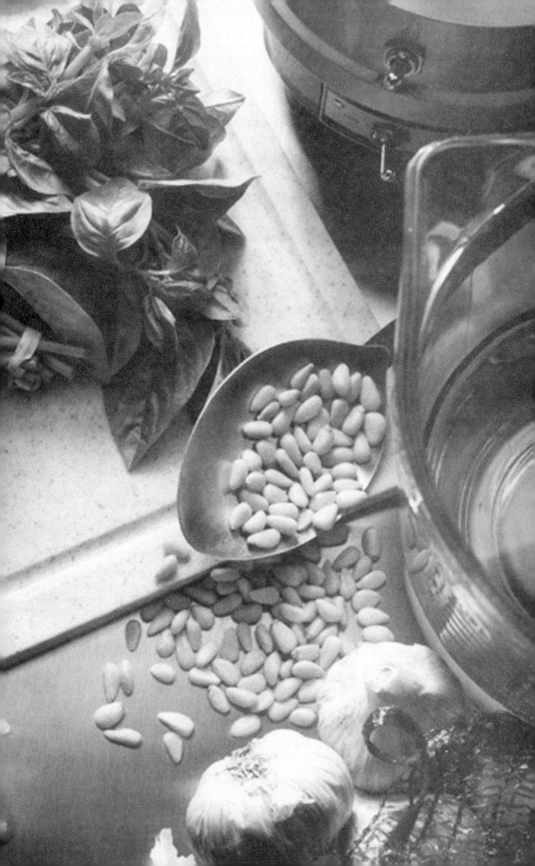

On the Side

The thing about side dishes is that they can be easily made into an entrée. Casserole suppers are so satisfying and delicious. How many times have we said, "Oh my, this tastes better the second day!"

When you feel this way about a recipe, you might want to double it when making it. Take the extra and set it aside in the refrigerator. Before serving for another meal in a day or two, add chunks of cooked meat, chicken or turkey, cover and heat until steamy and you have a quick, healthy and tasty casserole which is a one-dish meal.

An important part of getting fit and maintaining a healthy lifestyle is not only making it easy but satisfying. Side dishes are an opportunity to get creative and spice it up to your own desires. Take advantage of seasonal ingredients that are just picked or new on the shelves at the grocer. If you are shopping at a farmer's market, ask the grower for some ideas on how to make something healthy and delicious.

Many natural grocery markets will offer healthy side dishes that are ready to serve or heat and serve. Find some favorites and make *these* dishes your *fast food!*

Do not overlook the side dishes when going out. Often times you will find you can make a meal of a shrimp cocktail and some sautéed or grilled vegetables. Add some rice or a baked potato and you have an inexpensive and satisfying meal.

FIT FOUNDATION tip

ingredients

Toasted Brown Pineapple Rice

1	tablespoon vegetable oil
2	eggs, lightly beaten
1	tablespoon fresh minced garlic
1	tablespoon fresh minced ginger root
2	bunches scallions
2	tablespoons sesame seeds
4	cups cooked brown rice
1	tablespoon soy sauce or to taste
2	cups fresh chopped pineapple
1/4	cup fresh chopped cilantro

directions

You may add leftover cut up cooked meat, poultry or seafood to this recipe and make it a one dish meal.

■ In a well seasoned wok or large heavy non stick saute pan over high heat, swirl the oil in the pan until hot and scramble the eggs in the pan until brown. Chop into small pieces and remove to a heat proof plate and set aside. Replace the pan to the heat and add the garlic, ginger, scallions and sesame seeds. Stir fry for a minute or two and add the rice to the pan. Stir fry while drizzling the soy sauce over the pan and stir fry until the rice begins to crisp on the edges, about 5 minutes. Reduce heat to medium and stir in the egg, pineapple and cilantro. Stir fry for 30 seconds just to mix. Serve immediately.
Serves 6 to 8.

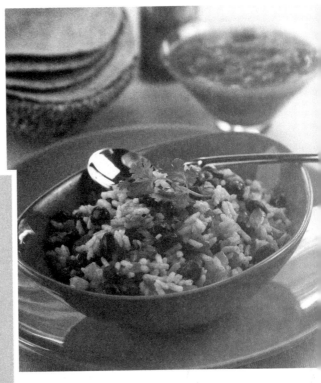

ingredients

Pinto Beans and Rice

16	ounce can pinto beans
8	ounce can corn kernels
2	tablespoons canola oil
1	medium sweet onion, peeled and chopped
1	green bell pepper, seeded and chopped
2	cups cooked brown rice
1	tablespoon low sodium soy sauce
1	tomato, seeded and chopped
1	tablespoon mild chili powder
1	tablespoon ground cumin

directions

The addition of grilled chicken or lean pork makes this a perfect, healthy and high protein meal.

■ Drain the beans and the corn in a colander. Heat the oil in a large sauté pan or Dutch oven over medium high heat. Stir the onion and pepper into the oil and sauté until tender. Add the cooked rice to the pan and drizzle the soy sauce over the top. Sauté the contents of the pan for 2 or 3 minutes and add the tomato, chili powder and cumin. Reduce heat to medium, stir to mix well and add the drained beans and corn. Cook until the beans and corn are hot.

Serves 4.

On the Side

107

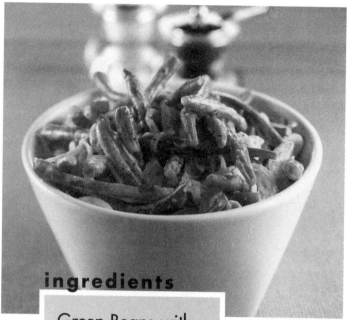

ingredients

Green Beans with Toasted Almonds

1	pound green beans
1	tablespoon butter
3/4	cup sliced or slivered almonds
1	teaspoon soy sauce or to taste
1	teaspoon ground black pepper

directions

■ Trim and rinse the beans. Boil in salted boiling water until tender, drain and rinse under cool water to stop the cooking process. In a large sauté pan or Dutch oven, heat the butter until it begins to bubble and in it sauté the almonds until they begin to toast. Working quickly, add the soy sauce and pepper to the pan and then the beans. Sauté together just until the beans are hot. Serve hot.

Serves 4 to 6.

ingredients

Tuscan Marinated Mushrooms

2   tablespoons vegetable oil
16   ounces small, similar sized mushrooms, baby bellas, white or oyster, trimmed and rinsed
$\frac{1}{8}$ cup vermouth
1   teaspoon dried Italian herb blend
$\frac{1}{8}$ cup extra virgin olive oil
1   tablespoon balsamic vinegar
Salt and pepper to taste

directions

■ Heat the vegetable oil in a heavy non-stick sauté pan over medium high heat and in it sauté the mushrooms for 5 minutes. Drizzle the vermouth over the pan and then stir in the herbs. Sauté until there is little or no liquid left in the pan. Remove from heat and cool to room temperature. Drizzle the mushrooms with olive oil and vinegar and season with salt and pepper.

Serves 4 to 6.

directions

■ Mash ingredients except tomato together while using the back of a fork. Now stir in the tomato. If you would like to refrigerate before serving, cover with plastic wrap with the top touching the entire top of the guacamole to prevent any air from affecting it, which will cause it to turn brown. Alternatively, you may frost the guacamole with salsa.

Makes about 2 cups

ingredients

Spicy Guacamole

3   medium sized rip avocados
Juice from 2 fresh limes
1   small minced onion
1   jalapeño pepper, seeded and minced
1   tablespoon cumin powder
1   teaspoon mild chili powder
Hot pepper sauce to taste
1   tomato, seeded and chopped

On the Side

ingredients

Roasted Red Peppers

4	red bell peppers
2	tablespoons olive oil
1	teaspoon fresh minced garlic
1	tablespoon soy sauce
1/2	cup crumbled blue cheese
3	tablespoons balsamic vinegar
1	teaspoon dried Italian herb blend

directions

■ Trim, seed and quarter the peppers. Place in a zipper lock bag with the oil, garlic and soy sauce. Shake to coat the peppers. Grill the peppers over medium hot coals (they may also be broiled) until charred and evenly blistered. Place back in the zipper lock bag and seal for a few minutes. Remove the skins from the peppers and discard (I often grill them just until tender but not completely charred and leave the skins on for this salad). Arrange the peppers on a serving platter and sprinkle the cheese over the peppers. Drizzle the vinegar over the peppers and dust with the herbs.

Serves 4 to 6.

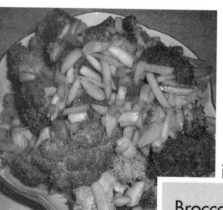

directions

■ In a large, heavy sauté pan over medium heat, place the oil and when hot, add the garlic and almonds and sauté for a minute or two. Add the broccoli and soy sauce and sauté another 2 minutes. Now add the vermouth and sauté until the broccoli is tender, another 2 or 3 minutes.

Serves 4

ingredients

Broccoli Almond Sauté

2	tablespoons olive oil
6	cloves garlic, thinly sliced
1/2	cup slivered almonds
4	cups chopped broccoli
1	tablespoon soy sauce
1/4	cup extra dry vermouth

ingredients

Pecan Rice Dressing

2	cups pecan halves
1	tablespoon olive oil
1	teaspoon salt
4	ounces butter
2	bunches scallions, trimmed and chopped
1	cup fresh minced parsley
1/2	cup fresh minced basil
1/2	teaspoon dried oregano
8	cups cooked brown or wild rice blend

Salt and pepper to taste

directions

■ Toss the pecan halves with the oil and salt and place in a single layer on a cookie sheet. Place in a pre-heated 375-degree oven to just toast, about 7 to 10 minutes. Remove from oven and place pecans in a heatproof bowl. In a large heavy skillet or Dutch oven over medium high heat, melt the butter and sauté the scallions until toasted. Stir in the herbs and the rice. Stir in the toasted pecans. Add salt and pepper to taste. Serve or place in a casserole and keep in a warm oven up to 90 minutes, loosely covered with foil.

Serves 8.

directions

■ Slice the eggplant into 1-inch thick slices and dip in the egg whites and then the crumbs to coat each slice well. Heat the oil in a large, heavy sauté pan over medium heat and in it brown the eggplant slices on both sides, in batches if needed and adding more oil as required. Drain on a paper towel lined tray. Place the sauce in the bottom of a 9 X 13 inch baking dish and place the eggplant in rows on top of the sauce, overlapping as needed. Sprinkle the cheese over the top. Bake in a preheated 350-degree oven until cheese browns and sauce bubbles.

Serves 6.

ingredients

Quick and Light Eggplant Parmesan

2	small similarly sized eggplants
4	egg whites, slightly beaten
2	cups seasoned bread-crumbs
3	tablespoons canola oil
3	cups tomato sauce
1/2	cup grated Parmesan cheese

On the Side

111

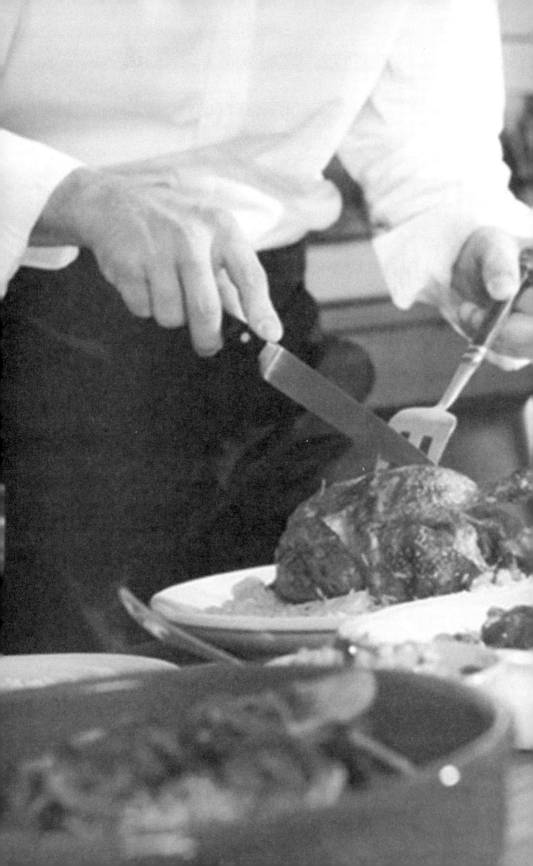

Entrées

When it comes to the main course, just about anything off the grill or roasted in the oven without a lot of fat will work. Try and make plenty so you will have leftovers that can save time when making the next meal or snack. I always say, "Today's grilled chicken breast is tomorrow's grilled chicken salad or quesadilla." Make it easy to eat healthy and get fit!

Skinless, boneless chicken is not only simple to work with, it is almost fat free and very high in protein. Turkey is the same. Both of these things are also very economical for large families. Fatty meats should be avoided. Try and choose foods that are all natural or organic. Stay clear of salty, nitrite laden preserved meats at all costs.

Cooking can be a time for family to be together having fun and getting creative. Make it a game to discover low fat delicious entrees that you can easily change and make over and over again. You'll find that not only is creating and eating healthy dishes is as simple as can be, it's fun!

Left over grilled lean meat or poultry makes an easy and accessible healthy snack. Cut it up and store it in a flavor-sealing container. Placed in the refrigerator next to some barbecue sauce for dipping and it is as inviting as it is delicious.

FITOUNDATION tip

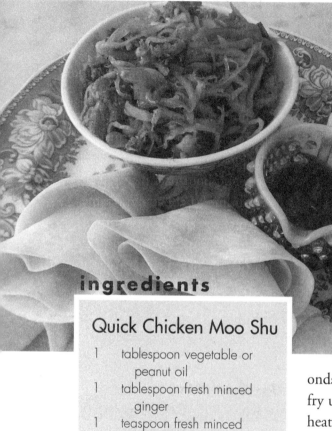

ingredients

Quick Chicken Moo Shu

1 tablespoon vegetable or peanut oil

1 tablespoon fresh minced ginger

1 teaspoon fresh minced garlic

1 bunch scallions, trimmed and cut into one half inch lenghts

1 cup shredded cabbage

4 cups cooked chicken, shredded

1 tablespoon sesame oil

1 cup Hoisin sauce (Asian section of grocery store)

8 to 12 small soft flour tortillas

directions

Additional Hoisin sauce and chopped scallions for garnish, if desired.

■ In a wok or large sauté pan over high heat, heat the oil and when it is hot, stir fry the ginger, garlic, scallions and cabbage for about 90 seconds. Add the chicken and stir fry until it is hot. Remove from heat and drizzle the sesame oil and hoisin sauce over the hot stir fry mixture and toss to coat everything with a glaze of the oil and hoisin. Serve immediately with warm soft tortillas or steamed Mandarin pancakes.

directions

■ Wrap the chicken breasts in plastic wrap and place in the freezer for 90 minutes. Place them on a cutting board and slice them as thinly as possible with a very sharp knife. Heat the oil in a large sauté pan or seasoned wok and stir-fry the chicken and carrots in the oil for 3 minutes. Add the garlic and ginger to the pan and stir-fry another 2 minutes. Drizzle the soy sauce over the pan and then sprinkle the sugar over the pan. Stir fry another couple of minutes. Add the scallions to the pan and sauté another minute or two. Serve immediately over rice or pan fried noodles.

Serves 4.

ingredients

Quick Teriyaki Chicken

3	skinless boneless chicken breast halves
2	tablespoons peanut or vegetable oil
1	cup shredded carrots
1	teaspoon fresh minced garlic
1	tablespoon fresh minced ginger
1	tablespoon soy sauce
1	tablespoon sugar
2	bunches scallions, trimmed, rinsed and sliced into 2 inch lengths; greens and whites

ingredients

Albacore Cakes

12	ounces fancy albacore tuna packed in water, drained
2/3	cup bread crumbs
1/2	cup toasted sesame seeds
1	teaspoon curry powder blend
1/2	teaspoon ground cumin
1/2	cup minced white onion
6	egg whites, slightly beaten
1	teaspoon Worcestershire sauce
2	tablespoons low fat mayonnaise
	canola oil for frying cakes

directions

■ Break apart the tuna with a fork and mix together with the bread crumbs and sesame seeds. Sprinkle the curry and cumin over the mixture and mix in. Stir in the onion, egg whites, Worcestershire and mayonnaise and mix well. Form 2 or 3 inch round cakes. Sauté in heavy, non-stick sauté pan or griddle over medium high heat using just enough oil to coat the pan. Brown for about 4 minutes per side, turning once.

Makes about 15 cakes, serving four to six.

Entrées

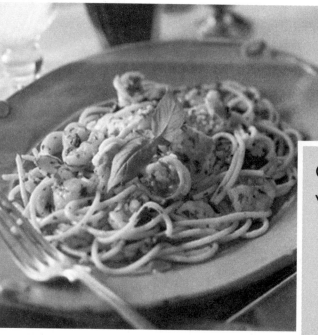

ingredients

Garlic Basil Pasta with Shrimp

1	pound fettuccine
1	teaspoon salt
2	tablespoons vegetable oil
1	tablespoon olive oil
3	ounces butter
3	cloves fresh minced garlic
1	green bell pepper, trimmed and cut into small pieces
1	tablespoon soy sauce
1	pound cleaned large shrimp, tails on
1	teaspoon sweet paprika
1	cup fresh rinsed basil leaves

Grated parmesan cheese as a garnish (optional)

directions

■ Drop the fettuccine into a pot of boiling water in which the salt and vegetable oil have been added and cook the pasta just until al dente, or slightly tough to the tooth. Drain well and toss the pasta with the olive oil. In a large sauté pan, melt the butter over medium high heat and stir in the garlic, green pepper, soy sauce and shrimp. Sauté until the shrimp are almost cooked, about 2 minutes, and stir in the cooked pasta and paprika. Sauté until the pasta is hot and shrimp are cooked and, just before serving, stir in the basil leaves. Serve immediately. Offer grated Parmesan cheese as a garnish, if desired.

Serves 4 to 6.

ingredients

Bow Ties and Barley

2	tablespoons olive oil
2	bunches fresh scallions, trimmed and chopped
2	red bell peppers, seeded and chopped
1	tablespoon dried Italian herb blend
2	cups pearled barley
1	tablespoon soy sauce
7	cups vegetable, chicken or beef stock
12	ounces small bow tie noodles

directions

■ In a large heavy skillet or Dutch oven, heat the oil and sauté the scallions and bell pepper until the scallions begin to toast. Add the herb blend, barley, soy sauce and stock to the pan. Bring to a simmer and simmer slowly until the barley is tender and all the liquid is absorbed, about 60 to 90 minutes. Boil the noodles until slightly tough, or al dente, and drain well. Stir into the barley. Raise the heat to high and sauté while constantly stirring the mixture just until it begins to brown. Serve or place in an ovenproof dish that accommodates the mixture and keep warm, covered or uncovered, for up to 90 minutes before ready to serve.

Serves 8 to 10.

Entrées

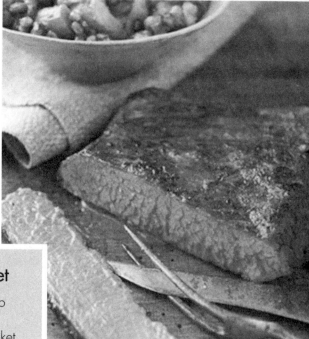

ingredients

All Night Beef Brisket

2	large onions, sliced into thick slices
1	5 to 7 pound beef brisket
4	cups water
2	bay leaves
2	cloves fresh garlic, sliced
1	tablespoon kosher salt
1	tablespoon fresh cracked pepper

directions

■ Arrange onions in the bottom of a high-sided roasting pan that will accommodate brisket. Rinse brisket and lay on top of onions fat side up. Pour water into pan and place bay leaves in water. Arrange garlic over the top and sprinkle with salt and pepper. Seal pan tightly with foil and roast in pre heated 275-degree oven overnight or 8 hours. To remove fat, chill brisket until fat hardens and remove. Slice or chop brisket and place in an ovenproof dish. Re-heat and strain juices and pour over brisket. Cover and heat to serve.

Serves 12.

ingredients

Turkey Fajitas

2	tablespoons olive oil
2	onions, cut into strips
2	cloves garlic, minced
1	red bell pepper, seeded and cut into strips
1	green bell pepper, seeded and cut into strips
1	tablespoon soy sauce
2	cups julienned turkey
1	tablespoon cumin powder
1	tablespoon mild chili powder

Juice from two fresh limes

6   medium soft flour tortillas

For garnishes: Shredded pepper jack cheese, guacamole, sliced black olives and salsa

directions

■ Place the oil in a heavy, non-stick skillet over high heat and in it sauté the onion, garlic and bell pepper strips for a couple of minutes. Drizzle the soy sauce over the vegetables and then add the turkey to the pan. Reduce heat a bit and sprinkle the cumin and chili powder over the pan. Squeeze the lime juice over the pan and then sauté another minute. Serve with the tortillas and garnishes of choice.

Serves 4.

ingredients

Pineapple Mustard Slow Cooker Chicken

2	red onions, sliced into thick rings
1	cup chicken broth

About 24 ounces skinless boneless chicken, cut into large chunks

1	cup prepared Dijon mustard
30	ounces pineapple chunks, drained

directions

■ Place the onions in the bottom of a slow cooker with the chicken broth. Toss the chicken chunks in a mixing bowl with mustard to coat. Arrange in even layer over the onion slices. Spoon the pineapple chunks over the chicken. Slow cook for 6 to 8 hours or until chicken is cooked to very tender. Serve over pasta or rice.

Serves 4

Entrées

Quick Orange Chicken

2   tablespoons vegetable or peanut oil

About 24 ounces skinles boneless chicken, cut into small chunks

2   yellow onions, cut into thin strips

4 or 5 cloves fresh sliced garlic

2   tablespoons fresh minced ginger

1 or 2 red bell peppers, seeded and sliced into thin strips

1   tablespoon soy sauce

1½   cups orange preserves

1   tablespoon fresh orange zest

directions

■ In a wok or large sauté pan over high heat, heat the oil and when it is hot, stir fry the chicken until it begins to brown and then add the onions to the pan. Stir fry another minute and then add the garlic, ginger, bell pepper strips and soy sauce. Stir fry for 1 minute and reduce heat to low. Stir in the orange preserves and zest and bring to a simmer. Make sure chicken is sufficiently cooked and serve immediately with cooked brown rice, if desired. *Serves 4*

directions

■ Brown the meat while scrambling constantly in a heavy, non-stick sauté pan over medium high heat. Meat should be very brown and dry, about 15 to 20 minutes. Stir in soy sauce, garlic and ginger and sauté 2 minutes more. Stir in sesame seeds and sauté 2 minutes more. Season with sesame oil. Remove from heat and stir in hoisin sauce. Take a head of iceberg lettuce and trim off the bottom. Remove as many whole leaves as you can, trimming from the bottom as needed. Rinse cups and drain on towel. Fill cups with warm filling and serve immediately. *Serves 4 to 6.*

ingredients

Lettuce Cups

2   pounds lean ground chicken, turkey or pork

2   tablespoons lite soy sauce

¼   cup fresh minced garlic

¼   cup fresh minced ginger

¼   cup sesame seeds

1   teaspoon sesame oil

¼   cup hoisin sauce

12-14   lettuce cups

shredded scallions for garnish

ingredients

Queso Fundido

1 lb.	lean ground pork
2	tablespoons fresh minced garlic
$1/2$	cup fresh chopped scallions
$1/8$	cup balsamic vinegar
1	tablespoon ground cumin
1	cup prepared black beans, rinsed and drained
2	poblano peppers-seeded and diced
2	mild green chilies-seeded and diced
1	cup shredded low fat Jack or Cheddar cheese
8	soft, fresh wheat tortillas

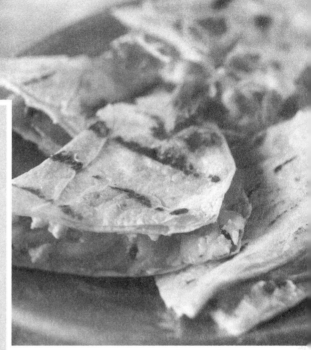

directions

■ Brown ground pork in a heavy, non stick skillet until very well done, scrambling constantly to break apart. Stir in garlic and scallions and sauté for a few minutes more. Add vinegar, cumin and black beans. Sauté. Add peppers and chilies. Sauté until peppers are tender. Turn heat to low and top with cheese and cook undisturbed until cheese is melted. Warm tortillas in microwave oven while cheese melts. Place a generous spoonful of meat filling in a tortilla and eat like a taco. Serve with low fat sour cream, shredded lettuce and chopped onions. A few sliced jalapeños will allow those who like it hot to heat it up!

Serves 4.

Entrées

ingredients

Fettuccine with Roasted Vegetables

1   head fennel, trimmed, rinsed
      and cut into strips
1   purple onion, cut into chunks
1   yellow zucchini, trimmed
      and sliced
1   red bell pepper, trimmed
      and sliced
1   green bell pepper, trimmed
      and sliced
2   tomatoes, trimmed, seeded
      and quartered
1   cup large pitted black
      olives, drained
1   teaspoon fresh minced
      garlic
2   tablespoons extra virgin
      olive oil
cracked pepper and kosher salt
      to taste
1   pound dried spinach
      fettuccine
salted water for boiling pasta
$1/2$ cup minced basil leaves
1   tablespoon minced oregano
      leaves
$1/4$ cup chopped Italian parsley
      leaves
shaved parmesan cheese as a
      garnish

directions

■ Toss the vegetables with the garlic and oil. Spread on a baking sheet and sprinkle with cracked pepper and salt. Place in preheated 325 degree oven and roast until fennel and peppers are tender, about 25 minutes. Just before vegetables are finished (they may be held in a warm oven up to 1 hour) cook pasta in boiling salted water until al dente. Drain pasta and toss with vegetables. Mix together fresh chopped herbs and sprinkle over pasta and vegetables. Serve with shaved parmesan.

Serves 4 to 6.

ingredients

Fish Tacos

4	6 ounce pieces of fresh haddock fillet
1	tablespoon Cajun seasoning
2	tablespoons olive oil
1	firm tomato, seeded and chopped
1	small purple onion, chopped
2	small mild green chilies (Anaheim), seeded and minced

Juice from 2 fresh lemons
| 1 | teaspoon ground cumin |
| 1 | tablespoon chopped fresh cilantro or flat parlsey |

Salt and pepper to taste
2	avocados
1	teaspoon soy sauce
12	steamed corn tortillas

directions

Serve these tacos and spicy guacamole with fresh sliced watermelon for a delicious summer supper.

- Rinse the fish fillets and drain on paper towel. Place on oiled parchment paper in roasting pan, pretty side down. Sprinkle the fish with Cajun seasoning and drizzle the oil over the fish. In a mixing bowl, mix together the tomato, onion, chilies, lemon juice, cumin, cilantro or parsley and salt and pepper to taste. Cut the avocado flesh into squares and mix into the salsa. Cover with plastic wrap and allow it to touch the top of the salsa. Place the fish on a middle shelf in the oven under a hot broiler and broil for 3 or 4 minutes. Turn the fillets and drizzle the soy sauce over the new side of the fish. Broil just until cooked and brown, another 3 minutes or so. Using a fork, separate the fish pieces into flakes on a warm plate and serve with salsa and the warm tortillas.

Serves 6

Entrées

123

directions

■ Discard or use for another purpose the neck and organs if included with the chicken. Rinse the chicken well, inside and out and pat dry with paper towel. Place on a rack in a roasting pan. Place the garlic and rosemary in the cavity of the chicken. Rub the skin of the chicken with the oil and sprinkle liberally with salt and cracked pepper. Roast in a pre heated 325 degree oven for 22 minutes per pound of chicken. The juices of the chicken thigh will run clear when the thigh is pierced with a sharp knife tip when cooked.

Serves 3 or 4

ingredients

Garlic Rosemary Roasted Chicken

1 whole roasting chicken
1 head garlic
1 ounce fresh rosemary
3 tablespoons vegetable oil
1 teaspoon salt
Cracked pepper to taste

directions

■ Mix together and marinate chicken or pork, cover and refrigerate up to 8 hours.

ingredients

Marinade for Grilled Chicken or Lean Pork Fillets

For 6 to 8 chicken breasts
2   cups white wine
$1/4$ cup olive oil
1   tablespoon soy sauce
1   tablespon fresh minced garlic
1   tablespoon dried Italian herb blend
1   tablespoon fresh rosemary leaves

directions

- Heat the oil in a 2 or 3-quart heavy saucepan over medium high heat and in it sauté the onion for about 5 minutes. Add the garlic. Sauté a few minutes more. Cut the veggie burgers into small pieces and add to the pan, Sauté while crumbling the burger pieces until the mixture resembles ground meat. Add the cumin and chili powder to the pan and mix it in well, sautéing another minute or two. Mix in the beans and keep warm. Heat the taco shells in a 300-degree oven until they are hot and toasted. Divide the taco filling among the shells and serve with the garnishes of choice.

Serves 4 to 6.

ingredients

Veggie Tacos

3 tablespoons vegetable oil
1 onion, peeled and chopped
2 cloves garlic, minced
4 veggie burgers
1 tablespoon ground cumin
1 tablespoon mild chili powder
1 can vegetarian refried beans
12 taco shells

Garnishes: shredded lettuce, salsa, sliced jalapeños, sour cream and chopped avocado.

Entrées

ingredients

Baked Swordfish and Brown Rice

2	tablespoons canola oil
1	tablespoon fresh minced garlic
1	onion, chopped
3	cups vegetable stock
2	cups brown rice
1/2	cup fresh minced parsley
6	1-inch thick 8 to 10 ounces swordfish steaks
	Juice from 3 lemons
2	yellow and 2 red tomatoes or 4 red tomatoes
1	cup fresh basil leaves
1/2	cup fresh chopped scallions
2	tablespoons extra virgin olive oil

directions

Toasted pine nuts for garnish (optional)

- Heat canola oil in a heavy saucepan with tight fitting lid over medium high heat and in it sauté the garlic and onion until golden. Add the vegetable stock and bring to a boil. Stir in rice and cover. Reduce heat to allow for simmer. Simmer 40 minutes or until rice is tender and liquid is absorbed. Remove from heat and fluff with fork. Cool rice. (You may successfully substitute quick cooking brown rice.) Stir parsley into rice. This step can be done the day before.

- Place the rice in the bottom of a baking pan or dish that will accommodate the fish in an even layer. Rinse swordfish steaks and place on top of the cooked rice. Squeeze lemon juice over the fish and rice. Core and slice tomatoes and arrange attractively over fish steaks and scatter basil leaves over that. Sprinkle with scallions and drizzle with olive oil. Bake uncovered, in pre heated 350 degree oven until fish is cooked, about 20 to 25 minutes. Sprinkle with toasted pine nuts before serving, if desired.

Serves 6.

ingredients

Grilled Swordfish with Chili Cilantro Chutney

4	8-ounce swordfish steaks
1/8	cup lite soy sauce
1	tablespoon canola oil
1	teaspoon fresh minced garlic

Juice from 1 lemon
Fresh cracked pepper to taste
2 tablespoons sesame seeds

directions

■ To Grill Swordfish: Rinse and pat dry the fish. Place fish flat in a deep platter or casserole dish. Mix together the soy, canola, garlic, lemon juice, pepper and sesame seeds and pour over fish. Lift fish to allow marinade to flow under the pieces. Allow to marinate for 30 minutes. Grill over medium hot coals until just done, about 4 minutes per side for 1 inch thick steaks. Remove to warm serving platter and top with Chili Cilantro Chutney.

Serves 4.

directions

■ Trim, seed and chop the chilis. Heat oil in a non-stick sauté pan over medium high heat and stir in chilies, garlic and scallions. Sauté until toasted, about 6 minutes. Cool. Place in a bowl and mix in cilantro. Mix together the lime, honey and salt and pepper to taste. Drizzle over contents of bowl and toss to combine.

ingredients

Chili Cilantro Chutney

3	mild green chili peppers (Anaheim)
1	tablespoon canola oil
1	teaspoon fresh minced garlic
1/2	cup chopped scallions
1/2	cup cilantro leaves, chopped
1/8	cup fresh lime juice
1	teaspoon honey

Salt and pepper to taste

Entrées

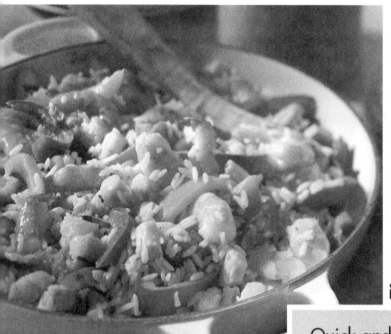

ingredients

Quick and Spicy Shrimp Jambalaya

2	tablespoons olive oil
1	chopped onion
12	ounces grilled or broiled spicy chicken sausage, cut into slices
2 to 4	tablespoons Cajun spice blend
3	cups cooked brown and wild rice blend
24 to 32	ounces zesty tomato sauce
16	ounces cooked large shrimp, tails on

directions

■ In a saucepan over medium high heat, heat the oil and sauté the onion until golden. Stir in the sausage and spice blend. Sauté for another minute or two. Stir in rice and tomato sauce. Bring to a simmer. Stir in cleaned and cooked shrimp just before serving. Cook only long enough to heat the shrimp. Serve with a soft tortilla.

Serves 4 to 6.

ingredients

Apricot Sesame Glazed Shrimp

For glaze

1	tablespoon extra virgin olive oil
3	minced shallots
1	tablespoon soy sauce
1/3	cup Cointreau
1 1/2	cups apricot marmalade
1/2	cup toasted sesame seeds

For shrimp:

Juice from 3 fresh lemons
2	tablespoons fresh minced garlic
1	tablespoon ground black pepper
1/8	cup light soy sauce
2	tablespoons extra virgin olive oil
2 to 3	pounds large or extra large peeled and cleaned shrimp

Mix together marinade ingredients and pour over shrimp to be marinated. Marinate for no more than 30 minutes

To broil or grill and glaze Shrimp:
2 fresh lemons, cut into wedges

directions

For glaze

■ Heat oil in a heavy saucepan over medium high heat and stir in minced shallots. Sauté about 2 minutes or until tender. Stir in soy sauce and reduce heat to medium low. Add Cointreau and cook another minute. Add marmalade to pan and when liquified, stir in sesame seeds. Bring to a gentle simmer and allow to simmer for another minute. Keep warm until shrimp are ready for glazing. Makes about 2 cups of glaze, enough for 2 or 3 pounds of shrimp.

For Shrimp

■ Skewer shrimp as desired on bamboo skewers and cap each skewer with a wedge of lemon. Broil or grill shrimp until just cooked, about 2 or 3 minutes per side, depending on size of shrimp. Remove to a warmed serving platter and pour warm glaze over shrimp as desired.

Serves 8 to 12.

Entrées

ingredients

Fast Fajitas

2	tablespoons canola oil
1	onion, peeled and sliced into strips
2	cloves fresh minced garlic
1	red bell pepper, seeded and sliced into thin strips
1	green bell pepper, seeded and sliced into thin strips
2	tablespoons soy sauce
1 to 1 1/2	pounds large cleaned and cooked shrimp, trimmed of tails
1	teaspoon ground cumin
1	teaspoon mild chili powder

8 to 12 fresh, soft flour tortillas
Guacamole, salsa and chopped lettuce for garnish

directions

- In a large, heavy non-stick skillet over medium high heat, place the oil and in it sauté the onion for about 2 minutes. Add the garlic and bell peppers to the pan and sauté another 2 minutes. Reduce heat to medium and drizzle the soy sauce over the vegetables and cook another minute or two. Turn heat to high and add the shrimp. Sprinkle the cumin and chili over them. Sauté until shrimp are sizzling hot. Serve with warm tortillas.

Serves 4.

ingredients

Teriyaki Grilled Salmon

2	tablespoons fresh minced garlic
2	tablespoons fresh minced ginger
$1/3$	cup maple syrup
$1/8$	cup light soy sauce
1	cup pineapple juice
2	tablespoons canola or extra virgin olive oil
1	piece salmon side fillet, skin on, about 24 to 30 ounces
$1/2$	cup brown sugar

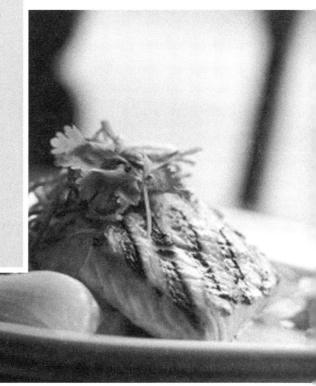

directions

- Whisk together the garlic, ginger, syrup, soy sauce, pineapple juice and oil. Pour over fish and let stand 20 minutes. Grill flesh side down, covered, over medium hot coals for about 5 minutes. Turn and sprinkle with brown sugar. Grill until done, about 6 to 10 more minutes, depending on thickness of salmon. Fish should be flaky and subdued in color when cooked.

Serves 4.

Entrées

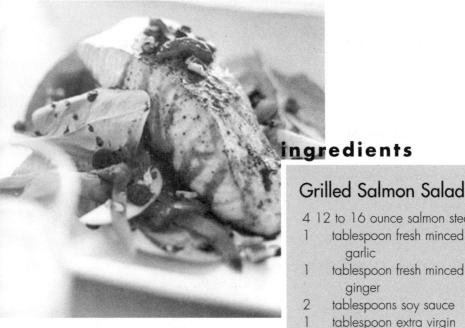

ingredients

Grilled Salmon Salad

4	12 to 16 ounce salmon steaks
1	tablespoon fresh minced garlic
1	tablespoon fresh minced ginger
2	tablespoons soy sauce
1	tablespoon extra virgin olive oil
1/3	cup capers, drained
2/3	cup snipped or fresh chopped dill
1	medium red onion, minced
Juice from 2 fresh lemons	

directions

■ Place the salmon steaks in a zipper lock bag with the garlic, ginger, soy sauce and olive oil. Shake to coat and allow to rest for 10 to 15 minutes. Grill over medium hot coals until just cooked, about 4 minutes per side for an inch thick steak. Remove from grill to cool, and then chill. Remove meat from skin and bones and place in a mixing bowl. Break apart meat into small flakes. Toss gently with capers, dill, and onion. Drizzle lemon juice over mixture and toss gently one more time to distribute juice. Let rest for 15 minutes and serve stuffed into a hollowed out tomato, over greens or with toasts. Or, cover and refrigerate up to 48 hours until ready to serve.

Serves 4 as a salad and up to 12 as an appetizer.

ingredients

Smoked Salmon Roll with Kefir Wasabi Sauce

1	English cucumber
16	slices smoked salmon
18	large fresh basil leaves
16	thin strips orange bell pepper
16	fresh chives pieces, each about 4 inches long

Kefir wasabi sauce (see below)

directions

■ Peel the cucumber, split it in half and remove the seeds. Using a mandolin or very sharp knife, cut the cucumber into very thin strips (fine julienne). Arrange a slice of salmon on a work surface. Place a basil leaf at one end. Place a small bundle of the cucumber strips on top of the basil leaf and place a strip of the pepper and a chive in the middle of the bundle. Roll up the salmon so that the cucumber is in the middle, sticking out of the top with the chive sticking out of that. Repeat with the remaining salmon and ingredients. Serve by standing upright on a pool of the Kefir Wasabi Sauce.

Makes 16 appetizers serving 8.

Kefir Wasabi Sauce

8	ounces kefir cheese or sour cream
1	tablespoon fresh minced ginger
1	teaspoon wasabi powder
1/4	cup soy sauce

directions

■ In a small mixing bowl, whisk all ingredients together until smooth.

Makes about 1 cup.

Entrées

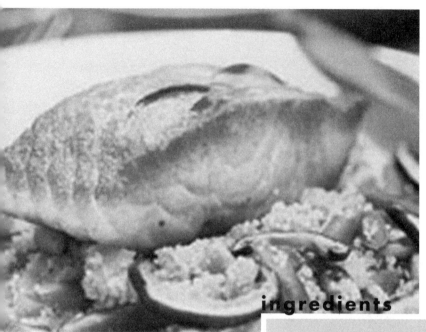

directions

Toasted sesame seeds for garnish (optional)

■ In a heavy non-stick skillet over high heat, place the oil and sauté the onion for about 1 minute. Pan should be *very* hot. Place the salmon in the pan skin side down and quickly mix together the champagne, ginger and soy sauce in a bowl. Pour over the salmon and cover immediately. Reduce heat to medium and poach the salmon until done, about 5 or 6 minutes depending on the thickness of the fillets. Remove to warm plate and dust with sesame seeds.

Serves 4.

ingredients

Ginger Poached Salmon

1	tablespoon olive oil
	A few thin slices of onion
4	6 to 8 ounce salmon fillets
1	cup champagne
2	tablespoons fresh minced ginger
1/2	teaspoon soy sauce

ingredients

Quick Garlic Sesame Shrimp

2   tablespoons canola oil
2   cloves minced garlic
1   tablespoon fresh minced ginger
1   bunch scallions, trimmed and chopped
1   red bell pepper, trimmed, seeded and chopped
1 to 2 pounds cooked cocktail style large shrimp, shelled
1   teaspoon light soy sauce
1/4 cup sesame seeds

directions

■ Heat the oil in a wok or sauté pan and stir fry the garlic and ginger for a minute or two. Add the scallions and bell pepper to the pan and stir fry another minute or two. Add the shrimp to the pan and then drizzle the soy sauce over the contents. Add the sesame seeds and stir to coat. Stir fry just until the shrimp are hot. Serve over cooked rice. Serve immediately.

Serves 4 to 6.

ingredients

Skillet Supper

2   tablespoons olive oil
1   24 ounce top sirloin boneless steak
1   baking potato, scrubbed and cut into cubes
1   red onion, chopped
1   green bell pepper, sliced
1   tablespoon lite soy sauce
1   beer
1   cup beef stock
cracked pepper to taste

directions

(The alcohol in the beer cooks out but it helps tenderize and flavor the meat.)

■ Heat the oil in a heavy non-stick skillet over high heat and brown the meat well on both sides. Reduce heat to medium low and remove meat from pan. Stir in potatoes, onion, bell pepper and soy sauce. Sauté for 1 minute and form a ring around the side of the pan with the vegetables. Leave the center of the pan free in which you will place the meat. Set the meat in the center of the pan and pour beer and beef stock over the pan and sprinkle liberally with pepper. Cover and cook over medium heat for 15 minutes. Turn meat, sprinkle again with pepper, cover and cook over low heat for 45 to 60 more minutes or until meat and vegetables are cooked and tender.

Serves 4.

Entrées

135

directions

■ Heat the oil in a large, deep, heavy non-stick sauté pan and sauté the garlic for 1 minute. Add the chicken and heat it in the oil while sprinkling the herbs and soy sauce over the pan. Stir in the spinach and as it begins to wilt, stir in the cheese. Serve immediately.

Serves 4.

ingredients

Greek Chicken

1   tablespoon extra virgin olive oil
1   teaspoon fresh minced garlic
4   grilled chicken breasts sliced thinly
1   tablespoon dried Italian herb blend
1   tablespoon soy sauce
8   ounces fresh baby spinach
1   cup crumbled feta with sun dried tomatoes and basil

ingredients

Asparagus Tofu Stir Fry

2   pounds young asparagus, trimmed and rinsed
1   gallon salted boiling water
2   tablespoons vegetable oil
1   tablespoon fresh minced garlic
1   tablespoon fresh minced ginger
1   teaspoon soy sauce
1   cup fresh chopped scallions
12 ounces extra firm tofu, sliced into 3/4 inch slices and browned in a small amount of oil in a hot skillet on both sides, cut up into small chunks
1/4 cup teriyaki sauce
chopped peanuts, toasted sesame seeds for garnish

directions

■ Place asparagus in a heat proof colander in the sink. Pour boiling water over to blanch. Cool under cold water. Cut into bite sized pieces. In a wok or sauté pan, sauté together the oil, garlic and ginger for 2 minutes over medium high heat. Stir in soy sauce. Toss in asparagus, scallions and tofu. Stir fry 2 minutes. Remove from heat and stir in 1/4 cup teriyaki sauce. Garnish with chopped peanuts and toasted sesame seeds.

Serves 6 over rice.

ingredients

Hoagies

for 1 hoagie:

1	6 to 8 inch long hoagie roll
1	grilled chicken breast, chilled and sliced
3	thin slices firm but ripe tomato
6	thin slices English cucumber
1/4	cup shredded carrot
1/4	cup shredded lite jack cheese
1/2	cup fresh organic baby greens
1	tablespoon extra virgin olive oil
1	tablespoon red wine vinegar
1/2	teaspoon fresh minced garlic (optional)
1/2	teaspoon dried Italian herb blend

salt and pepper to taste

directions

■ Using a serrated knife, cut a 'v' down the top of the roll to form a valley and reserve the created 'top'. Remove a good deal of the 'heart' of the roll. Fill with chicken, tomato, cucumber, carrot, cheese and greens. Mix together the oil, vinegar, garlic, herbs and season with salt and pepper. Drizzle over greens and replace 'top'. Wrap tightly in plastic wrap and keep cold until serving.

Entrées

137

ingredients

Day Before Shrimp Gumbo

2	tablespoons extra virgin olive oil
1	cup chopped celery
1	cup chopped onion
1	cup extra dry vermouth
1	cup fresh minced parsley
$1/2$	cup fresh chopped basil leaves
$1/4$	cup fresh chopped sage
2	tablespoons fresh minced tarragon
1	teaspoon fresh minced rosemary leaves
2	tablespoons fresh minced oregano
2	tablespoons paprika
84	ounces crushed tomatoes
2	bay leaves
2	tablespoons granulated sugar

salt and pepper to taste

2	cups fresh chopped or frozen okra
2	pounds freshly cooked, cleaned shrimp (any firm, cooked seafood will do)

2 to 3 cups cooked brown rice

directions

■ Heat the oil in a heavy stockpot over medium high heat and stir in the celery and onion and sauté until golden. Add vermouth and reduce heat to medium. Stir in parsley, basil, sage, tarragon, rosemary, oregano and paprika, Sauté 1 minute or so. Stir in crushed tomatoes and bay leaves and bring to a simmer, stirring frequently. Stir in sugar and season with salt and pepper. Simmer gently for 1 to 3 hours. To serve: add okra, shrimp, and rice to simmering gumbo and serve when shrimp is hot.

Serves 8 to 10

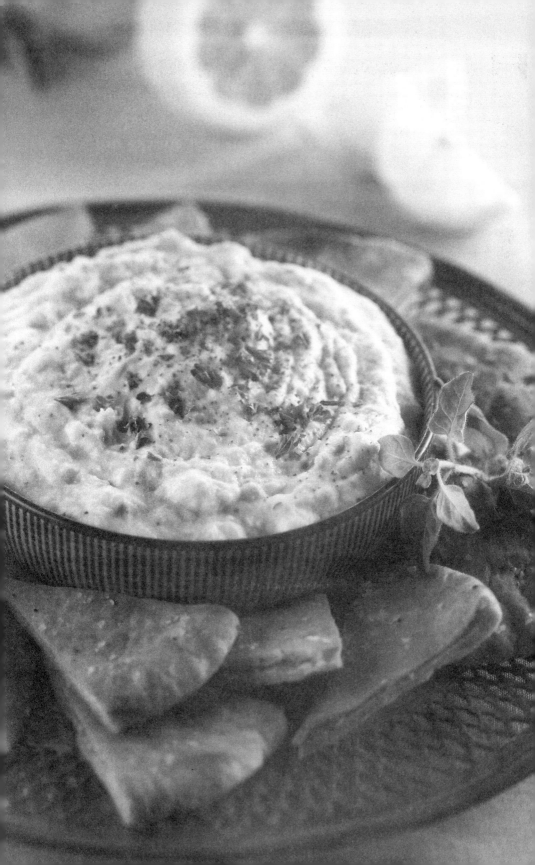

Snacks

There is a pre-conceived notion that snacks are **bad for you.** While it is true that *unhealthy* snacks should be avoided, a healthy snack between meals can not only give you a burst of energy but will reduce your hunger and intake for the next meal, which is a good thing. The key is finding a healthy snack assortment that you enjoy. Stay away from high fat, fried things and go toward the fresh choices. Crunching some celery and carrots or enjoying a crisp tart apple will *never* hurt you. A chilled, roasted chicken drumstick is perfect after school. Have grape tomatoes washed and ready to pop in your mouth. Slice a pear and dip it into fat free vanilla yogurt. Get crackin'! Do some snackin'!!!

Many people say not to ruin your appetite with a snack before a meal. To that I say "Ha!" Eat a personal watermelon an hour before a supper. Enjoy carrots dipped in hummus before lunch. Go ahead. Ruin your appetite with a healthy snack!

FIT FOUNDATION tip

ingredients

Baked "Fried" Chicken Fingers

4	skinless boneless chicken breast halves, cut into 1 or 2 inch wide strips
2	cups low or nonfat buttermilk
4	egg whites, slightly beaten
2	cups flour
1	cup crushed corn flakes
1	teaspoon garlic powder
1	teaspoon sweet paprika
1	teaspoon cracked pepper
	cayenne pepper to taste
1	teaspoon salt (optional)

directions

■ Preheat oven to highest setting. Place chicken in a bowl with the buttermilk and allow to stand for 30 minutes. Drain the chicken and place in the egg whites. Blend together the flour, corn flakes, garlic powder, paprika, peppers and salt. Place in a deep plate. Dredge the chicken pieces in the flour mixture to coat well. Place on a baking sheet or broiling pan that has been sprayed with cooking spray and place in hot oven. Reduce heat to 350 degrees and bake until done and crisp, about 25 to 35 minutes depending on size of chicken pieces. Juices of chicken will run clear when chicken is cooked and meat will have no pink coloring whatsoever.

Serves 4.

directions

■ In food processor, process cream cheese, cilantro, olives and cumin until smooth. Spread onto tortillas and roll up. Cut at an angle into inch wide slices.

Makes 18 snacks serving 6.

ingredients

Jalapeño Cheese Rollups

8oz.	low or nonfat cream cheese, softened
1/4	cup fresh cilantro
5oz.	jalapeño stuffed olives
1	teaspoon ground cumin
3	fresh wheat tortillas

ingredients

Low Fat 7-Layer Dip

1	can no-fat refried beans
1/4	cup dry-roasted sunflower kernels
1	cup guacamole
1	cup no or low fat sour cream
1	cup salsa
1	cup shredded low fat cheddar cheese
1	3.8-ounce can sliced black olives, drained (optional)

directions

■ On a deep plate, spread the beans in an even layer. Then, sprinkle the sunflower kernels over the beans. Spread the guacamole over that and then the sour cream followed by the salsa. Sprinkle the cheese over the top and then make a border around the plate with the olive slices. Serve with blue or yellow corn chips. Serves 8 to 12 as an appetizer. You may top the dip with cooked crab, shrimp or sliced chicken for a one-dish meal.

Snacks

143

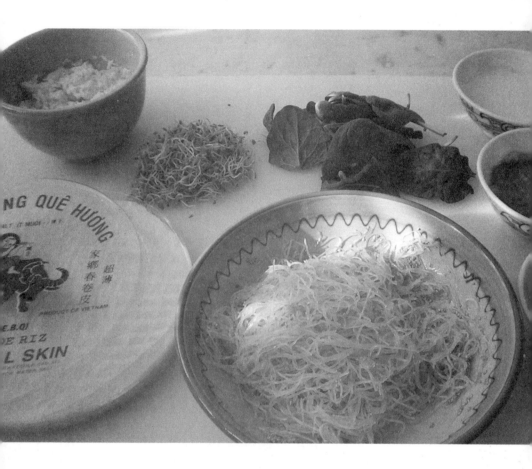

Fresh Spring Rolls

Sometimes you learn things in the strangest of places. My family and I enjoy fresh, Thai-style spring rolls that are full of fresh veggies, bean thread noodles and shrimp. Dipping sauces round out the equation and we can make a meal of them.

Going for a ride one Sunday afternoon, we saw a sign for Thai food in the window of what looks kind of like a

ingredients

Fresh Curried Crab Spring Rolls

24 large fresh basil leaves
2 cups prepared (see above text) chopped bean thread noodles
2 cups fresh alfalfa or clover sprouts
1/2 cup fresh chopped chives
1 cup fresh cooked crab meat mixed with 1/3 cup mayonnaise and mild curry blend to taste

ingredients

Fresh Shredded Chicken Spring Rolls

24 large fresh basil leaves
2 cups prepared (see above text) chopped bean thread noodles
2 cups fresh alfalfa or clover sprouts
1 cup shredded cooked and cooled chicken tossed with 2 tablespoons Hoisin sauce
1/2 cup fresh chopped scallion greens

biker bar. I think it best that I go in alone as my wife and daughter should wait in the car. Inside, this dreary and shabbily furnished place I see pleasant faces and smiles. I look at a menu and they have our craving and I figure I'd order them to go. Lucky for me, I was standing in front of the kitchen door as the chef prepared the spring rolls before my eyes.

It was the wrappers that puzzled me. I seem them in many super-markets and in Asian markets from coast to coast. They are called Spring Roll Skins. They are crisp sheets made of rice, salt and water. I have also seen the sweet-ened ones with coconut and other seasonings. But I didn't know how to get them from the crisp sheets to pliable, almost rubbery yet soft and workable.

There she was, this Asian chef,

Snacks

145

ingredients

Shrimp Spring Rolls

24	large fresh basil leaves
2	cups prepared (see above text) chopped bean thread noodles
2	cups alfalfa or clover sprouts
1	cup chopped, cleaned cocktail shrimp
1/2	cup chopped scallion greens

working quickly and efficiently on a large clean work surface, she dipped the sheets briefly in very hot water, placed them flat on the surface, filled them and rolled them up tightly. Brilliant! And, it couldn't have been easier. In a brief moment, she opened up a new culinary door for me and I am sure she was most unaware of it.

I have been making them at home ever since. One other curious ingredient that is traditional in these fresh blessed bundles of crunch is bean thread noodles. They are those almost clear bundles of threads that you see in the Asian section of many stores but may not know what to do with. Join the club. But again, once I learned, they have become a staple in my cupboard.

To prepare those, simply soak them for 5 minutes in hot water from the tap. Drain them. Cut in lengths as desired with kitchen shears and poach in boiling water for 30 seconds. Drain immediately and run under cold water to stop them from cooking. Drain them, and when they have cooled, toss with sesame oil and a bit of seasoned rice vinegar to taste until ready for use in the spring rolls. They also make a great side dish as they are in the sesame vinegar marinade with a dusting of toasted sesame seeds.

Now lets roll some spring rolls! Have all of your ingredients ready and then prepare a shallow dish with boiled water. The dish must be wide enough such that the spring roll skin can be laid on top of the water in a

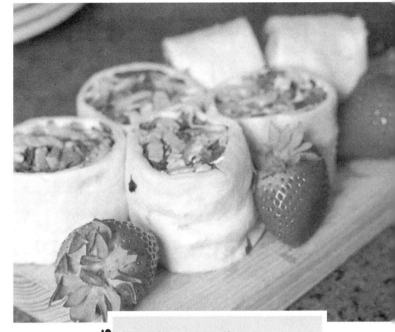

single layer, a heat-proof pie dish works perfectly as does a large sauté pan. Lay a skin on top of the water for 2 seconds and turn it over. Soak it for 2 or 3 seconds and lay it flat on a clean work surface. Place a large basil leaf or two in the center and a bundle of the filling ingredients over the leaves. Roll up tightly like egg rolls and place on waxed paper. Repeat for as many spring rolls as you intend to make. Cover and refrigerate up to 5 hours before serving. They should not touch each other or they can stick and tear.

For 12 fresh spring rolls, you will need about 6 cups of filling combinations. I have listed some of our favorites below based on using 12 skins along with some outstanding dipping sauces. And while these are great as a lunch or supper, they also make great do-ahead appetizers for your next party. You'll have your guests talking for days!

ingredients

Fresh Avocado Spring Rolls

24	large fresh basil leaves
2	cups prepared (see above text) chopped bean thread noodles
2	cups fresh alfalfa or clover sprouts
12	strips fresh avocado tossed in lemon juice
1/2	cup fresh chopped scallion greens

Snacks

ingredients

Peanut Butter Dipping Sauce

1/3	cup seasoned rice vinegar
1/2	cup chunky peanut butter
1	teaspoon soy sauce
1	teaspoon fresh minced garlic
1	tablespoon fresh minced ginger

directions

- Slowly stir the vinegar into the peanut butter until combined. Stir in the remaining ingredients until smooth except for the chunks of peanuts.

Makes about 1 cup.

ingredients

Scallions Hoisin Sauce

1	cup seasoned rice vinegar
1	tablespoon fresh minced ginger
1	teaspoon fresh minced garlic
2	tablespoons sesame oil
2	tablespoons toasted sesame seeds

directions

- Mix together and serve as a dipping sauce.

Makes about 1 cup.

ingredients

Ginger Wasabi Sauce

1	cup fat free mayonnaise
1	teaspoon ginger powder
Wasabi powder or paste to taste	

directions

- Blend ingredients together well.

Makes about 1 cup .

ingredients

Quick Pickled French Green Beans

8	ounces French green beans, trimmed and rinsed
2	tablespoons red wine vinegar
1	teaspoon or one cube turbinado sugar
$1/4$	cup chopped purple onion
2	tablespoons fresh minced dill

salt and pepper to taste

about 1 cup water

directions

■ Place beans lengthwise in an accommodating jar with tight fitting lid. Beans should be rather tightly fitting in jar. Pour in vinegar and add sugar, onion, dill and salt and pepper to jar. Add water to fill jar and seal. Shake jar to blend ingredients and refrigerate up to 3 days before serving. (Overnight works fine, too!)

Serves 4 to 6.

ingredients

Quick Spinach Herb Flatbreads

2	large spinach and herb flour tortillas, cut into 3-inch wide strips

Canola oil for brushing

directions

■ 'Paint' the strips of tortilla with oil and cook on griddle or on non-stick skillet over medium high heat until golden brown on both sides, turning once. Keep on paper lined tray in warm oven until all are toasted.

Serves 4.

ingredients

Herbed White Bean Hummus

1	can (15 ounces) prepared Italian white beans, drained and rinsed
1	teaspoon fresh minced garlic
1/2	cup fresh coarsely chopped basil leaves
	a few fresh oregano leaves
1/2	cup fresh chopped parsley leaves
	juice from 2 fresh lemons
1/4	cup extra virgin olive oil
1/2	teaspoon paprika
	salt and fresh cracked pepper to taste
	herbed crumbled feta cheese for garnish, optional

directions

- Place beans, garlic, basil, oregano, parsley and lemon juice in the bowl of a food processor fitted with a steel blade. Pulse to combine. Scrape sides and process just enough to blend. Add a bit of the oil to the bowl and then begin processing, adding the oil in a slow stream until desired consistency of hummus is reached. Season with paprika, salt and pepper. Refrigerate until serving. Bring to room temperature to serve. Garnish with feta and serve with flat breads, veggies or baked tortilla chips.

Makes about 2 1/2 cups.

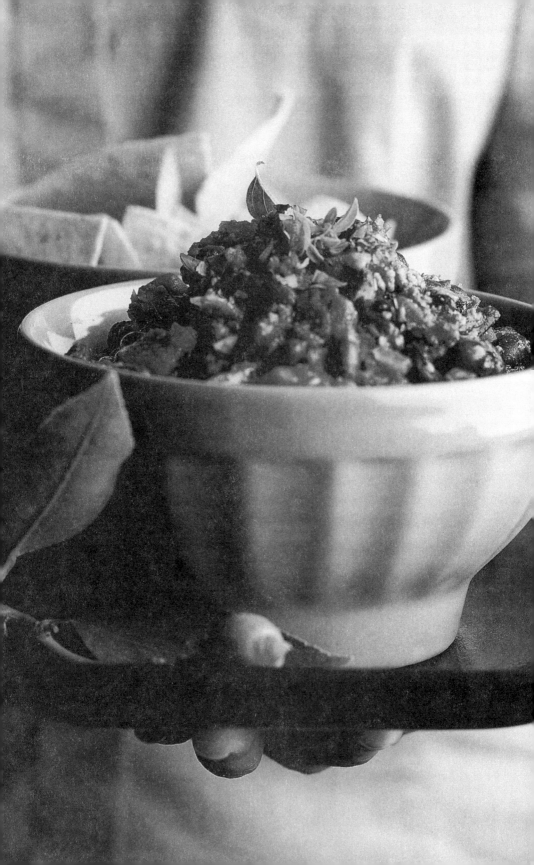

Salsas: All You Can Eat

That used to raise a red flag in the nutrition world. But there are things that can be eaten, even to excess, without a problem. And sometimes, when you have to munch, even for the wrong reason, there are choices you can make that will still keep you on the road to a Fit Foundation.

I thank heaven for salsa. The word salsa just sounds refreshing and zesty. A combination of crunch, spice and flavor that is more than just for chips. Salsa actually means sauce in Spanish. But most of us think of it as a cold, fresh chopped blend of ingredients.

And now, salsa has become a big part of menus and can be found accompanying all kinds of dishes from traditional tacos to roast chicken. Plus you are getting a serving of vegetables that kids will happily eat. It is a great choice instead of packaged high fat dips or nacho cheese sauce that is often times little more than colored and flavored hydrogenated oil.

With the following recipes, I have given some suggestions for serving. But let your imagination run wild. There is a salsa for every occasion!

Many of the salsa recipes that follow can also be served as a side dish for an entrée or served over greens for a flavorful salad. When it comes to salsa, make plenty!

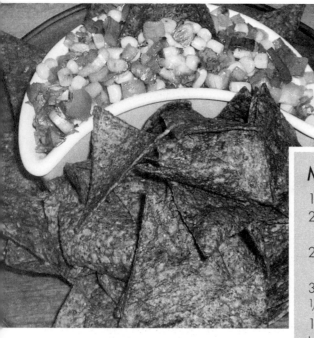

ingredients

Mango Lemon Salsa

1	small minced red onion
2	Anaheim or mild green chile peppers
2 or 3	jalapeño peppers or to taste
3	firm but ripe tomatoes
1/2	cup fresh chopped cilantro
1	mango
Juice from 2 lemons	
1/2	teaspoon ground ginger
1/2	teaspoon ground cumin
1/2	teaspoon sweet paprika
1/2	teaspoon chili powder

directions

This is wonderful with anything off the grill and with many curried dishes.

■ Mince the onion and place in a glass or ceramic mixing bowl. Seed the peppers (wear plastic gloves when handling the jalapeños!) and chop and add to the onion. Seed the tomatoes and chop them and add to the bowl. Coarsely chop the cilantro and add to the bowl. Cut the flesh of the mango into small cubes and add it to the bowl with the juice from the lemons. Add the ginger, cumin, paprika and chili powder. Mix well. Serve immediately or cover and refrigerate. Can be made up to 36 hours in advance.

ingredients

Avocado Salsa

1	small minced white onion
2	mild chile or bell peppers
2	firm but ripe tomatoes
1/2	cup fresh chopped cilantro
2 to 4	ripe Haas avocados

Juice from 3 limes
Salt and pepper to taste

directions

Wonderful as a veggie taco filling, with baked or organic blue tortilla chips, or served over greens as a salad. The avocado must be added to the recipe just before serving.

- Mince the onion and place in a glass or ceramic mixing bowl. Seed the peppers and chop and add to the onion. Seed the tomatoes and chop them and add to the bowl. Coarsely chop the cilantro and add to the bowl. Cut the flesh of the avocados into small cubes and add to the bowl with the juice from the limes. Mix well. Season with salt and pepper to taste. Serve immediately.

Makes 3 to 4 cups.

directions

This salsa is terrific with chips or with grilled chicken and shredded cabbage in a wrap sandwich.

- Mix ingredients together and serve.

Makes a bit over 2 cups.

ingredients

Quick White Salsa

1	cup chunky style all natural salsa from the jar
1	cup fat free sour cream
1	small chopped red onion
1	teaspoon ground cumin
1	teaspoon mild chili powder

Salsas

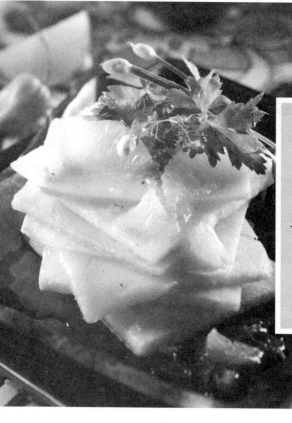

ingredients

Jicama Salsa

1	medium to large jicama
1	red bell pepper, chopped
1	bunch fresh scallions, chopped
Juice from 4 limes	
1	teaspoon chili powder
1	teaspoon ground cumin
$1/2$	cup shelled and salted sunflower seeds
Salt and pepper to taste	

directions

Jicama is a very healthy, high water and fiber content vegetable from south of the border. This salsa is great all by itself as a salad or side dish, besides being awesome with baked pita chips or "grilled" anything.

■ Peel the jicama and slice into thin slices. Then cut across the slices to form small squares of jicama. Toss together the jicama pieces with the bell pepper, scallions and lime juice. Sprinkle with chili powder, and ground cumin. Just before serving, stir in the sunflower seeds. Season with salt and pepper to taste.

Makes about 3 cups.

directions

Delicious with chips, over just about anything grilled, and with tacos and burritos.

■ If using fresh corn, boil the shucked corn in a solution of 1/2 skim milk and 1/2 water. Watch the pot to boil slowly to prevent boil-overs. It will take 15 to 20 minutes for the corn to be cooked. Drain. Brush corn with a bit of olive oil and grill or toast over an open flame until charred. Run a knife down the cob to remove the kernels. Place the kernels (fresh or canned) in a mixing bowl. Heat the oil in a skillet and roast the tomatillos in the skillet. Add the scallions to the pan and brown them a bit. Cool and place the tomatillos and scallions in a food processor and coarsely chop. Place in the bowl with the corn. Trim the tops off of the tomatoes. Using your index finger as a probe, remove the seeds and pulp from the tomatoes and chop. Place in the bowl with the corn. Add the cilantro, jalapeño pepper, lime juice and salt and pepper to taste. Mix well. Serve immediately or cover and refrigerate over night but do not add salt until just before serving as it will draw the moisture out of the vegetables and make a watery, wilted salsa.

Makes about 3 cups.

ingredients

Roasted Corn and Tomatillo Salsa

4 ears fresh sweet corn, shucked or one can corn kernels, drained
1 teaspoon olive oil (if using fresh corn)
1 tablespoon canola oil
6 firm tomatillos, paper-like skin removed
1 bunch scallions, trimmed, rinsed and chopped
2 to 3 firm but ripe tomatoes
1/2 cup coarsely chopped fresh cilantro leaves
1 jalapeño pepper, seeded and minced
Juice from 2 fresh limes
Salt and pepper to taste

Salsas

ingredients

Papaya Salsa

1	papaya, seeded and chopped
1	cup chopped red tomato, seeded
1/2	cup chopped cilantro
1	minced red onion
1	cup chopped mild green chiles

Juice from 2 medium limes
Salt and pepper to taste

directions

This is so wonderful with the Chilean sea bass tacos; I had to include the recipe below for the tacos!

■ Mix all ingredients together in bowl. Let sit for a couple of hours for flavors to fuse.

directions

■ Mix together the soy sauce, garlic, ginger and lemon pepper. Pour over fish and allow to stand for 15 to 20 minutes. Grill over medium hot coals until just done, about 5 minutes per side depending on thickness of fish. Remove from grill and cool. Fish should flake apart nicely. Divide fish pieces among warmed corn tortillas. Top with jack cheese. Serve hot with papaya salsa.

Serves 6.

ingredients

Chilean Sea Bass Tacos

1/3	cup lite soy sauce
1	teaspoon fresh minced garlic
1	tablespoon fresh minced ginger
1	teaspoon lemon pepper
12	ounces Chilean sea bass, bones removed, or other firm, white fish fillet
12	corn tortillas, steamed
1	cup shredded jack cheese

Papaya salsa

ingredients

Toasted Jalapeño Tomatillo and Watermelon Salsa

8 to 10 medium tomatillos (peel off parchment-like coating and rinse)
2 tablespoons vegetable oil
1 onion, minced
2 cloves garlic, minced
3 jalapeño peppers or to taste, seeded and chopped
1 tablespoon ground cumin
2 teaspoons mild chili powder
1 cup tomato sauce or purée
1 cup seeded watermelon chunks
Salt and pepper to taste

directions

■ Cut the tomatillos into quarters. Heat the oil in a large heavy sauté pan over medium high heat and in it sauté the onions for a few minutes and then add the tomatillos, garlic, and jalapeños. Sauté until the onions and garlic begin to brown. Reduce heat to low and sprinkle the cumin and chili powder over the pan. Stir in the tomato sauce and bring to a simmer. Remove from heat. Cool. Place in a blender or food processor with the watermelon and puree. Season with salt and pepper to taste.

Makes about 3 cups.

Salsas

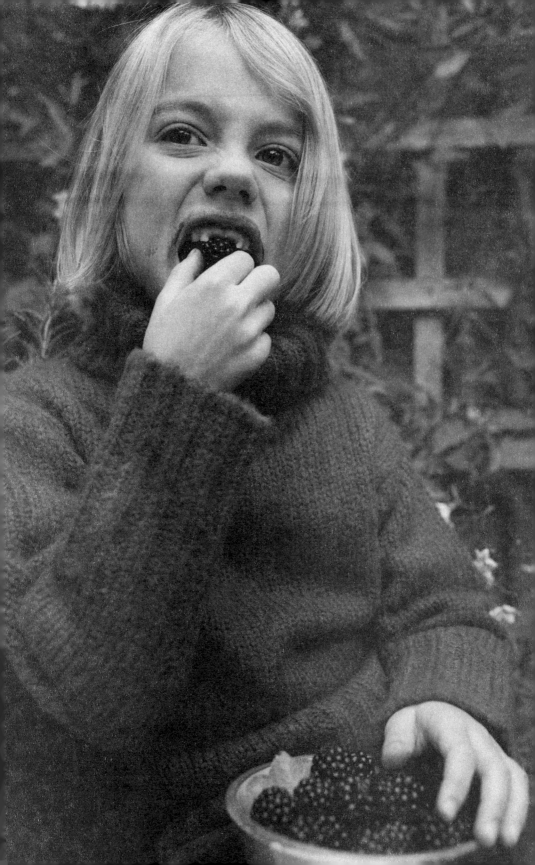

Sweet Stuff

I was on vacation with a large group of friends and family and we were staying in a resort. One of my relatives was a child who could not have been more than seven or eight and extremely overweight. Her father, who had never had or even understood what it was to have a weight challenge, made it his responsibility to get her skinny. She was allowed one "sweet treat" a day.

Earlier in the day she had enjoyed a homemade sweet bar that had enough calories to sustain an adult for a day. In the evening, we all gathered in the lobby for our last night together and it was decided that we would all have dessert.

When it was time for this precious child to order, she was interrupted by her father who proceeded to rudely remind her in front of everyone that she had already had her sweet for the day and that she absolutely could not have dessert. That poor child was expected to stand there and watch everyone else eat a sinfully rich

Fit Tip

The amounts of butter and sugars in some of these recipes are minimal when divided up by the number of servings. A little goes a long way when it comes to flavor and texture.

selection with her plate empty and her stomach yearning.

There were many choices for that child. First of all, her father had no business humiliating his daughter in front of everyone and making her feel embarrassed and different. He may have had good intentions but instead proceeded to basically punish and isolate her from the group.

What her father might have chosen to do was to quietly encourage his daughter to have a bowl of watermelon balls, a scoop of sorbet, or some frozen yogurt. He might have also taken her by the hand and personally walked her over to her grandparents or older relatives and asked them to share a story or bedtime tale to take her mind off of ice cream or cake. Another choice might have been to go to the gift shop for some window-shopping or even the purchase of a coloring book or post card.

It is important to take a positive approach and to make each child feel special for the gifts that they possess. To encourage and to reassure is the key, never to humiliate or embarrass. We all have choices to make. When we are making them for someone else, it is even more important to make the right ones. The effects can last a lifetime. Sweet stuff is not always a no-no.

ingredients

Blueberry Crumble

4	pints fresh blueberries
1/2	cup powdered sugar
1/4	cup unbleached all purpose flour

For topping:

4	tablespoons butter cut into pieces
1	tablespoon vegetable oil
1	cup oatmeal
1	cup unbleached all purpose flour
1	cup brown sugar
1/2	cup maple syrup
1/2	cup granulated sugar
1	teaspoon cinnamon

directions

■ Toss blueberries with powdered sugar and one-fourth cup flour. Place in buttered deep baking dish. Pulse topping ingredients in a food processor until the texture of coarse meal. Place in even layer covering berries. Bake in preheated 350-degree oven until bubbly and brown on top, about 35 minutes.

Serves 8 or up to 12 served a la mode with low or non fat vanilla frozen yogurt.

ingredients

Ginger Baked Apples

4	firm apples, cored
4	cinnamon sticks
8 to 12	whole cloves
10	ounces ginger ale
1/2	lemon
Dash	vanilla extract

directions

■ Place a cinnamon stick in the core of the apple and insert 2 or 3 cloves in each apple decoratively. Place apples in a deep baking dish with lid. Pour ginger ale over the apples and rest the lemon half in the center of the apples. Sprinkle a dash of vanilla over the apples and cover. Bake in preheated 325-degree oven for 90 to 120 minutes or until apples are soft but not mushy.

Serves 6-8.

Sweet Stuff

163

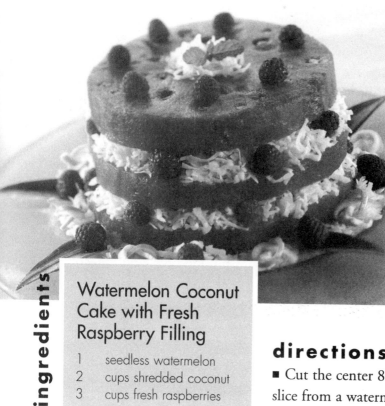

ingredients

Watermelon Coconut Cake with Fresh Raspberry Filling

1   seedless watermelon
2   cups shredded coconut
3   cups fresh raspberries

directions

■ Cut the center 8- to 10-inch slice from a watermelon. Lay it down on a flat work surface and cut around the rind and slide the rind off leaving a cylinder of watermelon. Slice into 3 slices as you would a cake. Place 1 slice of the melon cylinder on top of a serving platter. Surround it with a ring of coconut. Place 1/3 of the remaining coconut and 1/3 of the raspberries over the slice and repeat to form a 3-layer watermelon "cake." Attractively arrange raspberries and coconut on top. To serve, slice into wedges and present them upright.

Serves 8.

directions

■ In a heavy saucepan over medium heat, combine the berries and sugar. Bring to a simmer and simmer slowly for 10 minutes. Stir in cinnamon, vanilla extract and amaretto. Remove from heat and cool until just warm. Serve with slices of angel food cake.

Serves 12.

ingredients

Almond Strawberry Angel Cake

1	quart strawberries, rinsed and hulled
1/3	cup granulated sugar
1/2	teaspoon ground cinnamon
1	teaspoon vanilla extract
3	tablespoons amaretto
1	prepared store-bought or homemade angel food cake, sliced into 12 slices

ingredients

Quick Pumpkin Pie

4	cups fresh or canned pumpkin puree
1	cup brown sugar
1/4	cup maple syrup
1	teaspoon vanilla extract
1	pinch clove
3	eggs
1	prepared *Quick Ginger Pecan Pie Crust* (see page 168)

directions

■ Place the pumpkin, sugar, syrup, vanilla and clove in the bowl of a food processor fitted with a steel blade and process to blend well. Add the eggs and process just to blend in. Spoon into 1 Quick Ginger Pecan Pie Crust and spread attractively to make an even layer in the shell. Bake in pre heated 350-degree oven until set, about 45 minutes.

Serves 8.

Sweet Stuff

165

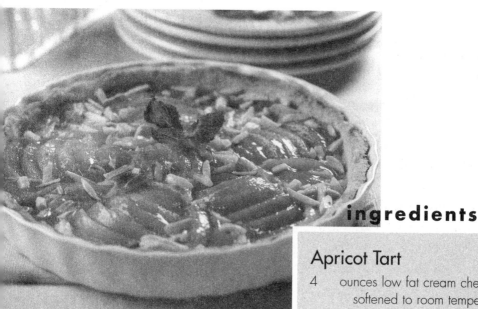

ingredients

Apricot Tart

4	ounces low fat cream cheese, softened to room temperature
2	tablespoons low fat sour cream
$1/2$	cup sugar in the raw
$1/2$	teaspoon vanilla
2	eggs, slightly beaten
1	baked 9-inch tart shell still in the false-bottomed tart pan
6	fresh apricots, pitted and sliced
$2/3$	cup apricot preserves
$1/2$ to 1	cup sliced almonds

directions

- Beat together the cream cheese, sour cream and sugar until smooth. Beat in the vanilla and eggs. Scrape mixture into the baked tart shell and smooth into an even layer over the bottom. Arrange the apricot slices attractively over the cream cheese mixture and bake in a pre heated 350-degree oven until the filling is set and starting to brown. Remove tart to a rack. In a sauce pan, melt the preserves and then brush the top of the tart to glaze. Remove the outer ring of the tart pan and paint the edge of the crust with melted preserves. Press the almonds around the preserve painted crust to create a border of almonds. Serve warm or at room temperature.

Makes 8 servings.

directions

- Place the dry ingredients in a mixing bowl. Whisk them together to blend well. Make a well in the center of the flour and put in the remaining ingredients. Beat at medium high speed for 5 minutes, scraping down the sides as needed. Pour into a greased 9 x 13 inch pan. Bake in a preheated 350-degree oven until it bounces back in the center when gently pressed with an index finger, about 40 minutes. It will be dark golden brown and just pulling away from the sides when finished baking.

Serves 8 to 12.

ingredients

Almond Honey Cake

2½	cups unbleached all purpose flour
1	cup granulated sugar
1	teaspoon baking soda
1	teaspoon baking powder
1	teaspoon cinnamon
1	teaspoon ginger
1	teaspoon ground nutmeg
1	cup ground almonds
½	cup strong coffee, cooled
½	cup Concord grape wine
¾	cup honey
½	cup vegetable oil
2	eggs
1	teaspoon vanilla extract

ingredients

Rice Pudding with Fresh Strawberries

4	cups cooked and cooled brown rice
1	can fat free sweetened condensed milk (14 oz.)
1	can skim milk (14 oz.)
3	eggs, slightly beaten
½	teaspoon cinnamon
½	teaspoon vanilla extract
1	pint strawberries, rinsed, patted dry and sliced

directions

- Cook over medium heat stirring constantly until slow boil is reached. Approx. 20 min. Remove to serving dish and cool. Refrigerate and just before serving, top with strawberries.

Serves 6-8.

Sweet Stuff

167

ingredients

Quick Ginger Pecan Pie Crust

For 2 Pies:

4 ounces pecan halves or pieces
8 ounces ginger snap cookies
4 tablespoons unsalted butter, cut into pieces
1 teaspoon ground cinnamon

directions

■ Pulse nuts and cookies in a food processor fitted with a steel blade until pulverized. Add butter and cinnamon and process until the mixture will hold its shape. Press into bottom and sides of two pie pans or dishes. Note: you can make the crusts in the food processor and then scrape out the bowl with a rubber spatula. No need to wash it before making the pumpkin pie filling. If you only need one crust, use one and wrap the other tightly and freeze for future use.

directions

■ Bake the cake according to directions, using over- sized muffin tins for baking, and cool. Rinse the raspberries and toss with granulated sugar and amaretto. Place in a saucepan over medium heat and simmer 10 minutes stirring occasionally. Place a shortcake on serving plate and surround with raspberry sauce. Sprinkle powdered sugar on top. Garnish with fresh raspberries.

Repeat for 8 servings total.

ingredients

Chocolate Raspberry Shortcake

1 organic chocolate cake mix
3 cups fresh raspberries
1/2 cup granulated sugar
1/8 cup amaretto
1/2 cup powdered sugar
Perfect raspberries for garnish

ingredients

Sweet Potato Plum Pudding

4 to 6 yams or sweet potatoes
6   tablespoons butter
1   cup maple syrup
Dash powdered clove
1   cup chopped pitted dried
    plums
Salt and pepper to taste
3   eggs, lightly beaten

directions

- Peel the yams and cut them into chunks. Gently boil the chunks of yam until tender and drain. Place them in a heatproof mixing bowl and mash the butter into them. Beat the mashed yams with maple syrup, clove, and salt. Salt and pepper to taste. Blend in the eggs and fold in the dried plums. Using a heat resistant spatula, scrape the mixture into a buttered shallow 2 to 3 quart baking dish and bake in a preheated 325-degree oven until puffed, golden and set, about 35 minutes. Serve hot or warm.

Serves 8.

Sweet Stuff

169

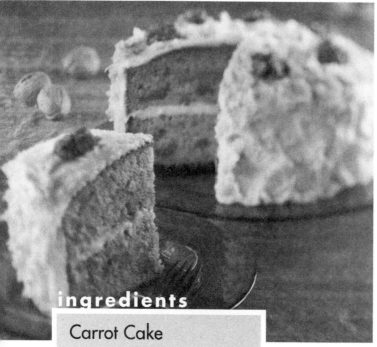

directions

- Place the flour, sugar, baking powder, baking soda, cinnamon and salt in a mixing bowl. Using a whisk, blend the dry ingredients well. Add the eggs, oil and carrots to the dry ingredients and stir to mix well. Stir in the vanilla. Divide the batter among 3 lightly oiled 9 inch round baking pans and bake in a pre-heated 350-degree oven for 30 minutes. Cool in pans for 15 minutes and turn out on racks. When completely cool, divide Pineapple frosting below between layers and on top of cake.

ingredients

Carrot Cake

2	cups unbleached all purpose flour
2	cups granulated sugar
1	teaspoon baking powder
2	teaspoons baking soda
1	tablespoon cinnamon
A	dash salt
4	eggs, slightly beaten
1 1/2	cups canola oil
3	cups finely grated carrots
1	teaspoon vanilla extract
1	recipe Pineapple Frosting- see following page

Serves 10.

ingredients

Pineapple Frosting

16	ounces fat free cream cheese
2	tablespoons softened butter
1	15-ounce can crushed pineapple, drained
2/3	cup powdered sugar
1	teaspoon vanilla

directions

- Bring the cream cheese and butter to room temperature. Meanwhile, drain the pineapple well and then place it in the center of a clean dish towel or double layer of cheesecloth. Roll the towel around the pineapple and twist from both sides to extract as much liquid as possible from it. Place the pineapple on paper towel. Beat together the cream cheese, butter, sugar and vanilla until fluffy. Blend in the pineapple.

Makes enough frosting for one 9-inch cake.

Sweet Stuff

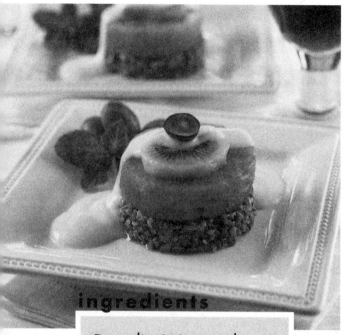

ingredients

Benedict Watermelon

1 1/2	cups low fat granola of choice
1/3	cup honey, room temperature
4 to 6	3-inch circles of seedless watermelon, 3/4 of an inch thick
4 to 6	half-inch thick slices of peeled kiwi fruit
1	cup low or nonfat creamy lemon yogurt
2 or 3	purple grapes, sliced into halves, seeded, for garnish

directions

This recipe is an incredible presentation and very easy to create.

■ Mix the granola with the honey by stirring as you drizzle the honey to distribute evenly through the granola. On a serving plate, make 3-inch circles of granola in even thickness, dividing the granola/honey mixture evenly among the servings. Top each of the granola circles with a watermelon slice and place a slice of kiwi on each watermelon circle. Spoon the yogurt over the kiwi and watermelon as though it were hollandaise sauce on eggs benedict. Top each watermelon benedict with a grape half, skin side up as a garnish reminiscent of the olive slice on eggs benedict.

Serves 4 to 6.

ALPHABETIZED INDEX FOR EACH CHAPTER

COMPLETE ALPHABETIZED INDEX